F***
You
Cancer

How to face the big C, live your life and still be yourself

***

Deborah James

Vermilion
LONDON

3 5 7 9 10 8 6 4

Vermilion, an imprint of Ebury Publishing,
20 Vauxhall Bridge Road,
London SW1V 2SA

Vermilion is part of the Penguin Random House group of companies
whose addresses can be found at global.penguinrandomhouse.com

Penguin
Random House
UK

First published by Vermilion in 2018

www.penguin.co.uk

A CIP catalogue record for this book is available from the British Library

ISBN 9781785042058

Typeset in 11/16.6pt Sabon LT Std
by Integra Software Services Pvt. Ltd, Pondicherry

Printed and bound in Great Britain by Clays Ltd, Elcograf S.p.A.

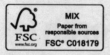

Penguin Random House is committed to a
sustainable future for our business, our readers
and our planet. This book is made from Forest
Stewardship Council® certified paper.

For Hugo and Eloise

'No time to turn at Beauty's glance,
And watch her feet, how they dance.

A poor life this is if, full of care,
We have no time to stand and stare.'

William Henry Davies

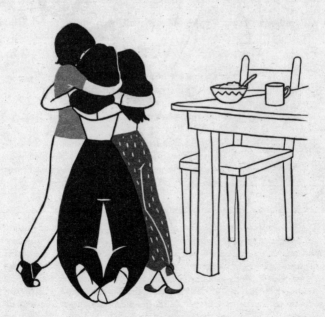

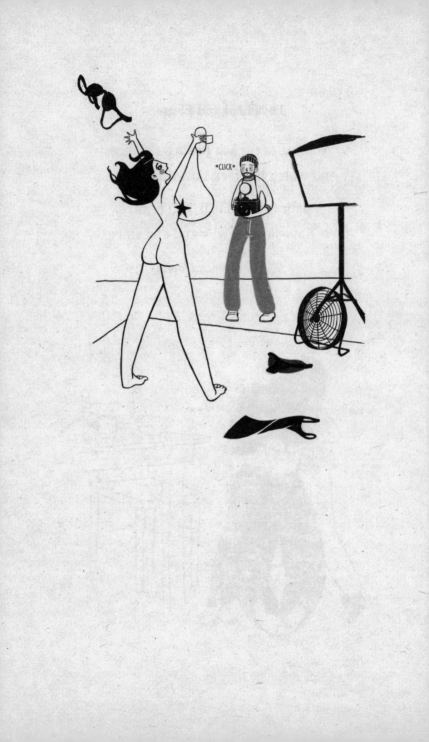

Contents

About the Author

Deborah James was a deputy head teacher leading national research teams into growth mindsets in schools. Then, in 2016, at the age of 35, she was diagnosed with stage 4 bowel cancer and her life with her husband and young children was thrown upside down. She's had four major operations, including bowel and lung resections, and multiple rounds of chemo, and is still undergoing treatment at The Royal Marsden Hospital. Rather than disappear into a cancer cave she started a blog, *Bowel Babe*, to debunk the myth that young women don't get bowel cancer, and writes a weekly column for the *Sun* online, 'Things Cancer Made Me Say'. She campaigns alongside major UK cancer charities, writes and presents the popular podcast 'You, Me & the Big C' for BBC Radio 5 Live and has built up a strong following on Instagram: @bowelbabe.

Chapter 1

It Was 6pm On an Idle Thursday

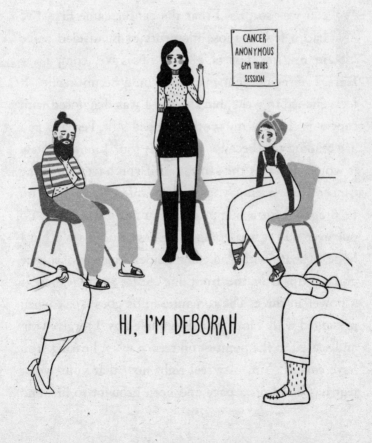

CANCER
ANONYMOUS
6PM THURS
SESSION

HI, I'M DEBORAH

My Name Is Deborah and I'm Not an Alcoholic

I too was surprised that the cancer came first. I've had a few of those moments of blindsided panic in my life, but of all my obsessive, compulsive fears, I never thought this one would be my reality. It feels clichéd to write, but the day I was diagnosed with cancer is the day my world stopped still. Perhaps you are reading this because yours has too? Life as I knew it would never be the same, and if you have joined the cancer club, a club you never wanted to be part of, be prepared for a bumpy ride. I'm not going to lie: no one ever said it was going to be easy, and it isn't, but I hope to share with you some golden nuggets of advice and top tips from the 'front line'. Some say that there is a power in three. The romantic in us goes weak when presented with 'I love you', is humbled by 'I forgive you' and scared to the point of no return when hearing 'You have cancer'. You may feel right now that your worst fear has lifted off a page and been brought to life, and you might not know how to put one foot in front of the other, let alone get your head around the idea of surgery or chemo. And I've been there – hell, I'm there right now, writing this not knowing what my next plan of action is, or what my pesky tumours are deciding to do. But the point is I'm finding my own way – with wine and high heels, shouting 'Fuck you cancer' as loud as I can as I prepare for yet another lung operation. It's not easy, and I don't know what my future holds, but I do know that when the big C enters, you can, with the right mindset, face it, live your life and still be yourself!

So, I've written this book to help you navigate the cancer rollercoaster in the knowledge that you are not alone. That's it's okay to have good days, bad days and everything in between, and that all those feelings you are experiencing are part of the ride, however crazy they may seem. But I'm going to give you a spoiler. I'm sorry to disappoint but I don't know the cure for cancer. I can't tell you if eating turmeric will help you, or doing 20 handstands a day will provide a cure. Trust me, I wish I knew.

But this is what I can tell you. I'm an average 36-year-old married mum of two. I was ploughing through life as a deputy head teacher, doing the 12-hour working days, trying to juggle kids, husband, friends, keeping fit, having a laugh and getting some sleep. I was on autopilot – my career took precedence, my relationships came last, dinner on the table would be considered a miracle and my kids gazed in disbelief if I ever actually turned up to something. I enjoyed the things many thirtysomethings do – wine, clothes, gossip, sex. I complained about lack of shut-eye, worried I wasn't 'making it' in my job, and was just about navigating the trials and tribulations that two crazy kids and full-time high-pressure jobs put on any marriage.

And then everything changed. On an idle Thursday, the week before Christmas, my worst nightmare became a reality. As I stared at my 6.5cm tumour during a colonoscopy, never did I realise more that the life I had been taking for granted would be the one thing I now desired above all else.

When I was diagnosed with bowel cancer, something only normally considered a possibility over the age of 60, my world spun out of control. As all cancer patients are, I was left to deal with a new life – one where my daily goal was to 'live', to get up and 'fight' cancer. But I'm human. You can't jump from a regular life to one of just trying to keep your head above the water without feeling like you are drowning at times. I had an outpouring of love, support and well-wishes but I was fighting to stay afloat. I had to find my own way through and find an element of control on an unpredictable ride, especially as the goalposts kept changing. And you will have to as well.

You may meet lots of people who will tell you that remaining positive, cutting sugar, eating a raw food diet or paying hundreds of thousands of pounds for an unproven nutrient drip will rid you of the beast that is cancer. 'You can beat it' they'll declare as you kindly hand over your hard-earned pennies in a quest for the holy grail of medicine. And perhaps it will work for you. I'm not a doctor, or researcher, and I'm not going to pretend I'm an expert in the field, because quite frankly I've met people who are and I feel totally humble in their presence. I've seen scientists kill breast cancer cells under the microscope with chemotherapy, which I took great pleasure in watching, but I've also listened to the brightest brains in the industry talk about just how clever even one little cell can be. If it wants to outsmart me or you it will – it doesn't matter how big or strong or ugly we are.

Doctors are, however, doing incredible things – and because of research, funding, technology and brilliant minds, today more people are living for ten years after the big C enters their life than die from it. But we are not there yet. We don't have a magic cure for cancer – but advances do mean that I've undergone procedures that a few years ago would not have been considered. It means I have a chance, and so do you. And with the right outlook you too can take control of a situation that might seem hopeless.

A cancer diagnosis isn't always game over – regardless of what the statistics might tell you. I was diagnosed with a cancer where stats told me only 34 per cent of women make it through the first year. Imagine celebrating a new year where you have a greater chance of dying than surviving! If I live to see my five-year cancer anniversary and my 40th birthday I will be one of only 9 per cent who do. But I'm not 'beating cancer', I'm just learning to live with it and navigating through the minefield it presents. I haven't done anything special that means I'm alive to write this today, and I pray for the sake of my kids that I can kick this can as far down the road as possible. But do I think I'll make it? Will I be there with fireworks, shouting 'Fuck you cancer' at my big four-zero?! Honestly – I'm not sure. While I believe in miracles, they work both ways, right? Hell, I'm the marathon-running, vegetarian-for-25-years, young woman who got the 'meat-eating, overweight old man' cancer.

As such, while someone is 'living' with cancer, I'm not convinced you have control beyond your mind and the way you deal with each challenge presented. That's why I created a character who was way cooler than me! 'Bowelbabe' – the alter ego I first started writing under in the early days – helped me believe that I could change the way I dealt with my diagnosis. She went further than I had ever imagined being able to, and I suppose hiding behind her positivity became my reality and showed me that I could live a fun life even while undergoing relentless treatment. She helped change how I perceived my cancer, and perhaps helped others to see how a life with cancer can look– and yes, it still included wine!

From this passion I wanted to share what I've learned, and am still learning, to help others know they are not alone. I wrote this for you – to give you strategies to deal with the tests presented. This book is not intended to tell you how to beat cancer or as a sob story memoir of what 'cancer taught me' – it's supposed to be your friend, your guide and your reassurance. It's the external voice that will tell you that it's okay not to be okay and that it's normal to laugh and sob uncontrollably all at the same time. It will not guide you through the intricate details of an MRI or CT scan, because there are hundreds of excellent resources provided by the wonderful charities I reference at the back of the book that will help you with that side of things. But it tells you the things you can't find in an information leaflet. The stuff that no one tells you, about how steroids might make you dance through the night, or how you cope with that dark dog of 'what if' – or how to find matching shoes to go with your chemo pump!

In a way I'm sorry you find yourself picking up this book – don't get me wrong, I'm thankful you did, but I'd rather you weren't in the club! However, now you've been initiated, I hope that you find the words comforting in your times of need, and uplifting (and funny) when you need a bit of a pick-me-up. You may be in the trenches, but let me take your hand and we'll be in this together. I'll be holding wine in the other hand; we can line up the cannons, rally the troops and send out a plane to sky-write 'Fuck you cancer' again and again in the hope it gets the message. Love Deborah x

Chapter 2

Welcome To the Club

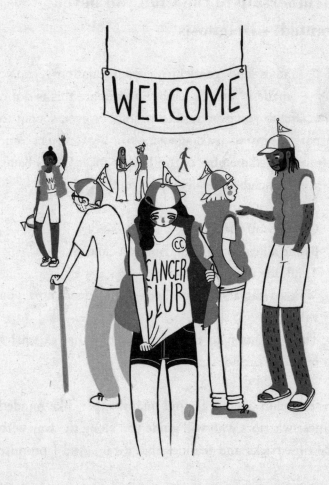

Membership of the Club you never wanted!– Diagnosis

Ladies and gentlemen, congratulations: you've made it into the club. I appreciate this is not a club you ever applied to join, or even sought to be part of – but with a diagnosis of the big C, you become a fully fledged member of the 'Fuck Cancer Club'. Being part of this club generally gives you the right to:

- Cry uncontrollably.
- Blame all irrational behaviour on cancer.
- Think life is unfair.
- Wax lyrical about how wonderful life is now you value it.
- Throw caution to the wind and buy that expensive handbag/car/holiday.

In the club you will find many other like-minded cancer warriors who will guide you along the way with the tips, tricks and realities that await. And I promise you – at 3am when the steroids kick in and you are pacing up and down your living room, they will be doing the same! You are not alone.

Living With Cancer

So, life does indeed go on – even if you have cancer on board! It may be a pain in the arse to drag it around everywhere with you, but unfortunately, while it's easy to become part of the club you never wanted to join, it's as difficult as hell to get out of it. You may, and I hope you do, become a cancer survivor. Someone who once had cancer, and it is now a distant memory of a difficult part of your life – but has at the same time defined every step you've taken since. You may, like me, have to learn to 'live' with cancer, knowing it might never leave but making the most of the days you do have. Either way, life can't be put on hold. I wrongly assumed when I was first diagnosed that I'd crawl into a black hole for six months, keep myself to myself, get my head down and sleeves rolled up, get through the treatment and put it all behind me. That I'd simply suspend my current life and, a little further down the line, pick up straight where I had left off – how much can really change in six months anyway? Oh how wrong I was!

Your New Life Has Begun!

Cheesy moment alert: I'm not one for loving it when people wax lyrical along the lines of 'Oh I'm so grateful to cancer for making me realise how important X,Y or Z is' – mainly because Cancer Is Shit. But I can't deny it's a wake-up call to life. Annoyingly, I'm sure that, like everyone who has ever had cancer, I'd much rather have checked into a week of 'sort your life out' rehab to give me that life-defining 'Oh wow' moment – but it wasn't to be. Instead I'm left having to live my life in the shadow of the big C, while feeling gutted that I might have to fit a lifetime of experiences into a much shorter timeframe. I was always known for working at 100mph but the stats I'm up against now just take the piss! Even on a steroid high, we are pushing it.

But this is the new normal. And perhaps, like me, you are still getting your head around the welcome pack to your 'new life', thinking how on earth do you balance all this and still smile? I'd hazard a guess that this 'life' probably doesn't look like the one you planned with your schoolmates in the playground aged ten, but after you wipe your nostalgic tears of mourning away, I promise you – with the right mindset you can still live a fulfilling life, and learn to make the most of everything. 'What, you take your chemo pump to the pub?' I'm often asked. 'Well yes. I also take it to the cinema, the theatre, on photoshoots and shopping – lucky chemo pump! For me this is a mindset that works – the 'I'm going to carry on as normal anyway' one. If you feel rubbish, of course listen to your body, curl up and chill – but if you feel okay, why should poison dripping into you stop anything? (within reason of course!).

A Work/Life Juggling Act

'Will you be juggling your chemo around work?' I was asked in my first oncologist meeting. I thought he was joking – 'People work on chemo?' I exclaimed with utter surprise. At this point I was getting in the rations and building the den, believing that I would only emerge from hibernation once it was all over. It soon became clear that the aim of treatment is not only to cure, or prolong your life, but to balance up a 'good quality of life' against the treatments' side effects. Perhaps it might not be the exact one you once had, but managing side effects effectively is key. I never expected that, on chemo, I would be taking holidays, having a laugh at parties and still exercising – albeit on my good days only. I thought everything stopped. That you went into a cancer hole, and came out as a dishevelled butterfly – or maybe a half-eaten moth is more accurate.

'But of course, you need to have things to live for,' said one of my doctors often, as I'd request for the fifth time to shift a chemo session so I could go on holiday. And yes, the show must (and can) go on.

Can I Still Work?

So, this is totally up to you and will depend on your financial circumstances, sick pay and the nature of your job, if you have one. I was working full-time in my role as deputy head teacher – which meant that I had to be totally reliable and if I didn't turn up, someone else would need to cover for me. This kind of role simply doesn't lend itself to an unpredictable treatment plan, when you are at the beck and call of your bloods being right, or hospital scans, or cancelled operations; I'd be letting the kids I taught down and that wasn't fair. So I took a break from teaching until I knew more about what my treatment might look like and how I'd feel.

However, something unexpected happened and I share it with you as a warning! Along with cancer came a mourning for the loss of my regular job, and life, for that matter. The job that I wanted to get up for every morning, the one that meant I could have hilarious conversations each day and feel like we were making a difference. I enjoyed the school community I worked in, the children I taught and the colleagues I shared laughs with even under pressure. Yes, I loved my job. While my school were incredible at reaching out to me when I got ill, I didn't feel part of the team any more, the one that was buzzing off each other on a daily basis. I had a huge gaping hole in my life that was being filled with cancer and only cancer. 'What are you doing today?' I'd think to myself, and the answer would be 'I'm doing cancer, urm, just trying to stay alive – again!'

Time to Fill the Gap!

The double whammy of cancer and a stop to my regular daily routine meant that I sometimes felt I didn't have a purpose. As my depression reached new heights, I needed to have something more than 'chemo' to live for – that doctor was right! Yes I know I've got two adorable monsters, and it goes without saying that they are my world, but I'd never been a stay-at-home parent. By four months on both of my maternity leaves I'd had enough of dirty nappies and the crying and had packed myself back off to work. I was a better mum when I could just shit in private – fact. But cancer meant I was around more, so I figured I'd better give the parenting malarkey a shot! My illness forced me to become a mum, albeit ten years down the line. Yes, my children are still rubbish at turning up with the correct stuff,

I hate bath time unless gin is involved, I avoid the school gate like the plague and I seem to have to de-nit my children more than I have to de-flea the bloody dog, but a part of me likes my recent attempts to stop my children becoming fucked-up screen-obsessed robots!

I then managed to throw myself into what seemed like an avalanche of varied projects. Alongside my number one job of being Mum, I was determined to share my story to raise awareness that if it can happen to me, it can happen to any one of us. I started a blog, which I used as my cathartic outlet. I fell in love with writing. I discovered a whole new online family and support network through social media. I was able to connect with people going through similar things to me and gain first-hand tips, tricks and other shoulders to cry on along the way. I started offering to write for other people's blogs as well as newspapers and before I knew it I had taken up an entire new career in broadcasting and journalism while undergoing my treatment – but there's nothing like a new challenge to keep you going, I'd convince myself while travelling to record another podcast in Manchester two days after an operation! I'm not advocating a total career change for everyone, but I am advocating keeping your mind busy at all costs. And not with cancer. The more you have going on, the less you have time to dwell and overthink your cancer. The more you can say 'Hang on cancer, I can't do you today because I'm busy', the easier the days when you do have to 'do cancer' will be. Have open and honest conversations about your job, negotiate how your role can be adjusted to accommodate your treatment and try to keep an element of your life before cancer going. If it's not work it might be weekly outings, seeing friends, attending a book group or visiting the local National Trust park or property. Either way, keeping a routine that's far removed from cancer is just as important as keeping your hospital and treatment routine.

Playing the Cancer Card

Congratulations! You have been given a cancer card – possibly the only positive of cancer. Now use it well and use it wisely. Unless you have some kind friends with a laminator prepared to actually knock one up for you, the 'cancer card' is an invisible pass, and it's granted to anyone with cancer to essentially 'Blame Cancer' for their actions. Be warned – your friends and relatives might get a little bored of you using it, and if you try to blame your pre-cancerous traits on cancer it really will be game over. It goes without saying that you should use the card when you are genuinely feeling too tired to do something, but don't use it when you are just trying to avoid your in-laws, in case they then see you down the pub with your mates on a Sunday afternoon enjoying the unlimited Prosecco brunch offer ...

Try using it to:

- Get out of any household chore – EVER.
- Buy that handbag you've always wanted.
- Debate with the ticket attendant when he fines you for that double yellow line parking.
- Get a plane or train upgrade (if it works for you, please let me know how you did it).
- Get a free round of drinks or a candle on your pudding in a restaurant. When you are asked 'Are you celebrating anything special?' you can say 'Yep, another round of chemotherapy for my CANCER' and see if the drinks roll in (or not!)
- To get a quick reservation at a sought-after restaurant.

Celebrating Milestones

I want to highlight the importance of celebrating from the start. Coping with a cancer diagnosis, going through treatment and coming out the other side is reason enough to remind yourself at every opportunity just how brilliant you are. Even when you don't feel like you are, and you've totally lost sight of where you might find that superhero cape from again, remind yourself how bloody strong you are being – and don't justify it with 'Well, I have no other choice.'

But I'm going to let you into a secret. I used to get a bit annoyed when people would practically hold up signs or ring a bell saying 'Treatment done – I've beaten cancer.' Without a shadow of a doubt it's the green-eyed monster in me that is jealous and fearful that I might never be able to do that. There is also the pessimist in me that says 'Don't you want to wait a few years to make sure you're in the clear?' But then I get a grip and think – good for them; and good for you too when you get the opportunity to be at that point. You are showing the world how kick-arse you can be and that should be saluted! It's about celebrating the small things that really matter in life, not just looking for the big, blow-out finale of treatment; the one stage-fourers can only dream about. It's not about lowering expectations, but being realistic when cancer is coming at you full steam ahead.

It's recognising that just because there may not be a clear finish line in sight, every mile you cover is a goal reached, and a cause to celebrate. Just because the goal-posts might move along your journey doesn't mean you haven't already run a marathon and then some, and that should be recognised. So, pat yourself on the back, if you're like me buy that new lippy and have a glass of wine. Whether it's in celebration of your first cycle of chemo, your last, being a year down the line, or ten. Whether it's walking after an operation, or just getting the first good night's sleep, acknowledge your achievement in getting that far. It may not be the big milestone you want to be celebrating, but each small step will get you closer to that dream.

Life is a celebration in itself. Wake up each morning and be thankful you are here. I know that if you have been vomiting all night, it's certainly easier said than done and today you may not feel that grateful – but tomorrow is a new day!

Breathe – Time Out

You are going to need downtime. You may think you are an 100mph-type person but you will need to accept that 80 is still over the speed limit. It's hard to take time out if you are not used to it, but you don't want to end up like the *Titanic*, sunk because it was trying to show off. It's okay to be seen not to be doing everything – or anything, for that matter! There are no prizes for being the person who got through chemo without an afternoon nap. Make sure you build time in to take time out. It's important from the outset to know and listen to your body, as I suspect it's not quite the one you know from the past. I hear you that it's frustrating when you feel you need more naps than a newborn, but you have to remember your body will be going through a lot, so give it the rest and time out that it needs. It will enable you to shine on other days!

Get Some Headspace

Your headspace is just as important as physical switch-off. Shut everything down once in a while and get your mind off the cancer. Perhaps you can do this by reading a book, listening to some jazz or trying meditation to clear your mind. It's important to create moments of escapism. Moments where cancer doesn't get a look-in – even if it's just a grabbed hour here or there. For five minutes of every day try clearing your mind and focusing on your breathing. Allow nothing else to enter your mind beyond your breath. This is a great way to either start or end each day.

Invisible Illness – You Don't Look Like You Have Cancer

I generally totter on to the train in high heels, with a full head of hair and bright orange lips. It's hard to then request a seat in a packed carriage – unless I'm wearing my big shiny 'Cancer on Board badge', which, while being a lovely idea, simply doesn't match my outfits half the time! But without it, no one would offer up their seat for me – I don't look ill or pregnant and I'm not old and frail. But not only do my legs hurt more from standing than they used to, my balance is dodgy – especially in heels! The chemotherapy has made me wobbly like a jelly baby and I find myself wondering if everyone thinks I'm drunk at 9am as I fall into an angry-looking bloke – again …

I had a full on bitch-fight in the theatre toilet queue once. I had just had a bowel resection and when I had to go, I just had to go. Despite the fact that I have access to a RADAR key, which allows you access to accessible toilets up and down the country, I was literally hollered at as I ran to use the disabled loo: 'Oi, you don't need to use that!' shouted a lady in red. I exchanged two short words with her, words that you can find on the cover of this book. Half of me wondered if I should actually just shit myself to prove I was right, but then I figured the last laugh wouldn't be on me, more like all over me! But it did make me think long and hard about our idea of what cancer and other invisible illness 'looks like'. We do have a misconception in society that you need to be in a wheelchair, or walk around with a big badge declaring your illness, to be taken seriously. You may find yourself in situations where people question just how ill you actually are: 'You were all right to go to the theatre last night but you can't be bothered to meet us today?'

You do not need not justify your choice of how you spend your energy to anyone. People will eventually realise (although, sadly, you may have to remind them) that you have good days and bad days. And that, if you are all smiles and running around town one moment, you will more than likely pay for it the next day. Go easy on yourself – know there will be peaks and lows. Accepting that it's not plain sailing will enable you to build a tougher boat to weather the storm.

Your New Normal

Okay, so I'm going to allow you a small amount of time to crave your old normal – but then I ask you to draw a line under it and recognise that wishing things would just go back to how they were will only put you in a depressive tailspin. I appreciate I sound like a harsh head teacher at this point but I'm doing it for your own good! Step one in coping with your new life is accepting that this is now the definition of 'normal'.

It might mean having a brain that is slower and a body that doesn't function quite right – I mean, I'm 36 and right now I can't do up any bloody buttons due to numb fingers from neuropathy. I got so frustrated last night I actually ripped my shirt off. And not in a sexy way.

Your new life may mean never leaving the house without all your hospital numbers, or needing to get a new handbag (hidden positive opportunity here ladies!) to carry the sheer amount of 'just-in-case' medication you need to have on you at ALL TIMES. Going away is more hassle than taking a school trip of 80 children skiing (I should know), and will include blood thinners, hospital letters and a struggle to find an insurance company that seems like a mini court case. Perhaps your side effects will mean a walk outside in the winter will involve dressing for the Arctic to avoid any cold spasms, and 'going for a run' is really now just 'walking slightly faster than normal' in fancy sports gear.

But this might be your new life – and I hope for you it's temporary. Even so, it can be a good life. And hell, time is short, so we'd best make it a stonking one!

Hands in the Air Like You Just Don't Care

'Well Mummy, cancer sure seems like a rollercoaster, you better hold on tight,' said my ten-year-old when I first told him that Mr C was now part of the family. He could not have been more spot-on with his analogy. I look back at my life before cancer (BC). I thought it was stressful. I'd worry about not being a good mum, wife, deputy head. There weren't enough hours in the day to be good at anything, and anyway, I wasn't satisfied with just being good at something. I used to think that life was a rollercoaster of emotions – a big see-saw of good and bad days that you'd bounce through until hitting those moments when you are blindsided into understanding the fragility of life. I believe this more than ever now. There had been previous moments in my life when the world seemed unfair. When, for example, tragedy had struck my 18-year-old cousin out of the blue – she died in a car crash. It is then that you experience the lows, the anger and the frustration of unexplained events in your world. You dip big-time. However, by contrast, the birth of your children or that long-sought-after promotion fills you with the adrenaline to keep you floating through on a high – loving life and everything in it.

Cancer has the same highs and lows as a regular life, but in an intense and structured setting that leaves you for most part 'on edge', worrying about what might be. The beauty of 'real life' is not knowing when these lows and highs might happen; as such we can live a blissful existence for most of our days in the hope that most of our 'blindsiding' occurs on the 'happy' side of the spectrum. In cancer, each scan, each blood test, each chemo cycle could deliver with it news that will have you cracking open the Champagne with a cheer or sobbing into a whisky glass with fear. You can easily bounce from great news one day to hideous news the next.

So how do you cope with such an emotional head-screw? I don't pretend to have this cracked and later in the book I will explore this with you in more detail. But I suggest we set some simple ground rules – let's call them our cancer club 'House Rules' – as a starting point:

- Be kind to yourself – you are doing the best you can.
- Let go of the control freak in you, and hope for a bit of luck.
- Focus on controlling the life you can live today and making the most of the good moments.
- Know you don't always have to be brave – it's okay to be scared.
- Remember who you were before cancer and who you are underneath – you are still that person.

Just Tell Me it will be Okay

I wish I could – hell, I wish someone would tell me it would be okay too. But then Sod's Law says that good news will be followed by something else to be blindsided by. Recently, having had a positive scan result, I joked as my younger brother stood on the start line of the London Marathon that it would really suck if I beat cancer and he popped his clogs running the race. As I spent the night nervously holding his hand as he lay in a critical state in the resuscitation unit of a major hospital after he collapsed 100m away from the finish line, I was once again reminded that life doesn't go to plan – EVER.

We will explore mental health more in Chapter 8 but let's get thinking of some questions as a starting point. If you knew what was going to happen, would you stop living and enjoying it? Would you appreciate the highs without the lows? We need to accept that death and bereavement are part of life – all of our lives. By normalising the conversation around it we can start to live. None of us will know when our time is due to be up, but I suggest we don't spend the time we have, cancer-ridden or not, worrying about it and asking if it will be okay. Instead, we can leave that to the greater forces and hold on to stories of hope, of those who defy the odds, and to the special moments and people that make our lives today so rich.

By doing so, you will allow yourself the mental freedom to accept your cancer diagnosis – wherever it may take you. And yes, it's okay to be scared of the unknown – you'd be hard-pressed to find someone in 'The Club' who isn't scared. But that's okay – we've got your back.

Here my friend Steph Douglas talks about how her husband's diagnosis of cancer impacted on their lives and gives her best tips for coping when you become a member of the club:

We'd been married a couple of years and I was 14 weeks pregnant when I sat next to my 30-year-old husband as he was diagnosed with a rare thyroid cancer. To say it took the wind out of our sails is an understatement. He is still living with some traces of cancer – it isn't currently curable – but it hasn't grown since he finished radiotherapy seven years ago and we think and talk about it a lot less than we did.

Doug's diagnosis was a tough time – the toughest we've been through in 12 years – but one where we learned so much about each other and the people around us. Nothing like starting married life with a life-threatening diagnosis to keep the mind focused! I appreciate perhaps it's easy to see it like that because Doug is still here. Sometimes it helps with perspective; other times I still get annoyed about the shoes left in the middle of the kitchen. But it certainly taught us life is fragile.

We quickly learned that diagnosis is exhausting, and as tests and treatment generally aren't going to be over in a couple of weeks, anyone going through this needs to look after themselves. The patient, of course, but also the carer – to have the emotional and physical strength to support someone who has been diagnosed with cancer, they've got to be kind to themselves too.

Make Someone Else a Point of Information

Coming home from a gruelling day at the hospital and phoning round everyone with updates was too much, perhaps because I was pregnant and emotional anyway, and as information tends to change regularly. We assigned one person to be our sharer of updates among our friends and it really helped. Rather than worrying about communicating with everyone – and dealing with their reactions – we kept our friend in the loop and he passed it on. Same for both of our families.

Find Your Circle

I found I could stay strong for around three days and would then collapse a bit. I'd find my mind going to a dark place where I imagined Doug's funeral and I'd need someone else to pick me up. These are the same people who seven years on remember to ask how we're doing around the time of annual check-ups, and they are wonderful. Whether you need to talk about what's happening or you need the distraction of someone else's dramas – however mundane – there are some people who know exactly what to do and say and some who just don't. Don't feel obliged to see and speak to all the people who suddenly get in touch. We pulled up our drawbridge except to those who we really wanted to see and could be ourselves with, whether laughing or crying. The energy you have is too precious to waste on anyone else.

Accept Help

You don't need pitying looks and a head tilt. Someone who fills your freezer, tidies up without asking what needs doing or helps with lifts is invaluable. Now we have kids, I can see help with entertaining them would be a massive help for any families going through cancer.

Don't Buy Them Flowers ...

People want to show they care and if not local or in the inner circle, they often send flowers. It's a lovely gesture but if you're inundated with bouquets they can become another thing to care for when you're feeling pretty spent. As a friend going through cancer recently messaged me: 'My house looks like a fucking funeral parlour,' which is perhaps not the look anyone wants. For the Don't Buy Her Flowers website we developed the Stand Up To Cancer Care Package, working with the charity and some awesome women (including Deborah!) on what might be appreciated when someone is going through or caring for someone with cancer. Cancer is so personal, and what might offer comfort varies depending on many factors, so each package can be tailored from over 40 products, from COOK Food vouchers, ice lollies and G&Ts to cashmere socks and puzzle books. Five per cent of every package goes to Stand Up To Cancer www.dont-buyherflowers.com.

Welcome to the Club

TAKE-AWAY TOP TIPS

So now you've joined the club, here's a reminder of the key nuggets to focus on from this chapter that will help pull you through those first days of being newly diagnosed:

Tip 1 Life still goes on – and it can be a good one. Life doesn't end when cancer enters. It's just a new challenge for you to navigate.

Tip 2 Don't make cancer your number one thing 'To do' – work, hobbies, fun and friends all still come first.

Tip 3 Celebrate each and every milestone and realise you are doing brilliantly.

Tip 4 Take time out for yourself both mentally and physically.

Tip 5 Expect good days and bad days – cancer is a rollercoaster and you are in for the whole ride – but you can do this.

Just remember that although you didn't want to be part of this club, we've got your back – whether you like it or not! At times you may feel weak and you might feel like you can't do this. Your thoughts may take you into places of sadness – but just remind yourself:

• • •

'With the new day comes new strength and new thoughts.'

Eleanor Roosevelt

Chapter 3

Plans, Scans, Dots and Docs!

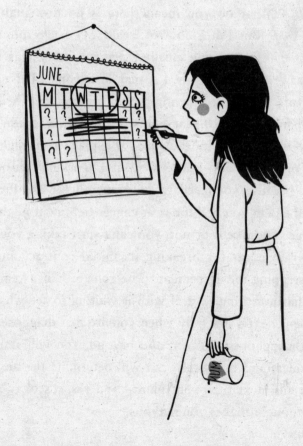

But I'm a Control Freak!

What do you mean there is no firm plan? But I'm a control freak! My background in teaching ensured that my diary was a military timetable planned a year in advance. I liked structure and I liked having a plan for my life – hell, I had five-, ten-, 20-year plans! Now cancer doesn't really like to play by the rules of a plan. You might start out with one – but let's call it a 'working' action plan, because you need to be prepared for the fact that the plan you had for your cancer treatment might change. And like it or not, you can't start taking your cancer to court for breaking its initial contract and overstepping the agreement to be gone in half a year! The hardest thing to deal with is waiting to see what happens next – not only when you are first diagnosed but throughout treatment and beyond. You will start to understand that each scan will determine the next steps and next treatment plan – and yes, it's okay if that thought makes you nervous.

What's the Plan?

You may have a very solid plan of, for example, 12 chemotherapy sessions, one operation and 20 radiation treatments. You may be able to see a clear end to your treatment and a date to work towards. You may have a clear plan that changes quickly – or you may be on a plan that says one scan at a time and we'll see what happens next. All of these options are normal; just be prepared to expect the unexpected – and yes, this can be in a positive way!

Shit Happens (Shock)

Did your world stop still the day you were diagnosed with cancer? Mine did. Life as I knew it would never be the same. Are you trying to compute the 100 different emotions that have flooded your brain the moment those words entered it? I recall shouting (well actually screaming) at the consultant who had just announced his findings – 'I don't want to die, please don't let me die' as I lay shaking in a hot sweat of blind panic, wanting to bolt it out of the hospital, run away and forget this ever happened. When I was younger I suffered from recurring night terrors; I'd wake up in a state of immense fear, imagining that I had a brain tumour and had just months to live.

I carried on living with heightened health anxiety through much of my teenage years and twenties, convinced the brain tumour would become a reality. Never, though, despite all my wild imaginary illnesses, did I think that bowel cancer at 35 would become my reality. And I bet you didn't think your cancer diagnosis would become yours either. Why me, I'd cry to my friends – well, why not you, I'd get in response!

Your Journey to Now

Draw a line under your journey to date and draw it now. A new one starts now your diagnosis is confirmed and it's healthier to focus on what's to come rather than dwelling on what might have been. Perhaps you are someone who is grateful for being diagnosed rapidly and at an early stage; or perhaps, like me, you have big regrets and are angry at how you arrived at this point.

Some people rock up at A&E and are diagnosed as they are being wheeled into the operating theatre, others come through standard screening programmes and others, like myself, get frustrated by a long-winded process of numerous GP visits, tests of exclusion and frustration over the hunt for answers. The actual cancer diagnosis, as scary as it might be, can be a relief – a confirmation that 'it wasn't all in my head' and the start of a plan of attack.

The Unknown is Scary!

After hearing the word 'cancer' my husband and I were silent in the car all the way home. I had what can only be described as uncontrollable tears streaming down my face. We immediately went to our local wine shop and proceeded to buy the most expensive bottle of wine on offer. We cracked it open, and then another, until I passed out in the hope that tomorrow things might be different.

Have you been pulled into a whirlwind of scans, tests and nervous waiting? The next day I was immediately whipped into scans, and within 24 hours I'd met the surgeon who was going to chop up my bowel a few weeks later. It's normal to still at this point be in a state of numb disbelief, as though you are not really in your body or hearing the barrage of information that is being thrown at you. It's fab to ask intelligent questions but it's also okay to simply nod as you are ushered to the next test – and yes, everyone jumps to the worst conclusion while waiting for results.

> Ensure someone else – a friend or relative – is always with you for all your initial tests and consultations. You may not be in the right headspace right now to digest the information thrown at you. Take along a notebook and get your friend or relative to write down key things said. You can then digest the details in your own time and think of, and write down, any questions you want answering by the team.

How Did This Happen?

'But I look okay.' And here lies one of the hardest aspects of the big C. Do you feel like you need to pinch yourself? Do I really have cancer? Maybe it's a mistake? Maybe they read the scans wrong? Hopefully I'll wake up soon and realise this is just a nightmare?

Personally, I had been justifying my symptoms as a product of 'modern life' and trying to have it all. As annoying as the symptoms were (blood in stools, weight loss, tiredness), I was still holding down a full-time job as a deputy head teacher, juggling the needs of two crazy kids and burning the twilight candle – hard. 'But I just ran 10K yesterday,' I pleaded with my consultant as he announced my cancer was stage four and I had tumours in both lungs.

Before you can accept the plan of attack, the diagnosis will need to sink in. Don't worry if you go into a dark place – a very dark place. For me that involved hiding in my bedroom for two weeks, googling the shit out of bowel cancer, not eating, drinking a lot of wine and refusing to get out of my pyjamas and get dressed. On the second week, my mum was at my house trying to coerce me into eating when a very blunt, wonderful friend popped round and was firm: 'Deborah, you really smell – I'm not leaving until you have got up, got dressed and are downstairs not attached to your phone.' Like a ten-year-old, I reluctantly obliged, and was then frogmarched out of the house to at least look at the sky and breathe in some fresh air for three minutes, before I felt overwhelmed and needed to hide again. The next day I went outside for five minutes, and slowly but surely baby steps brought me back to a functioning level – at least on most days.

There is no magic way you are supposed to feel or react when presented with those three words 'You've got cancer.' Everyone experiences a barrage of different emotions, perhaps only in the space of an hour.

And that's okay because I've learned another three words – 'You're not alone.'

It's okay to be deeply sad, relieved, scared and anxious all at the same time. It's okay to sob uncontrollably, to shout and scream that life isn't fair, to blame yourself, to blame others, to turn into yourself, to retreat and shut down communication. When you are first diagnosed, it's okay not to be okay.

Which Dot Am I? (Statistics and Prognosis)

Have you started googling yet? Are any of these questions familiar?

- What's my percentage chance of survival?
- Should I write my will now?
- Does turmeric really kill cancer?
- Am I going to die? – (yes I actually did type this into Google and it wasn't much help!)

I mean, there is cancer – the kind that is chopped out in ten minutes and you are back to work that afternoon – and there is CANCER. Don't get me wrong – any cancer can and does have a huge and wide-reaching impact on our physical and mental well-being – but should you really be worried if the statistics say that 99 per cent of people with your type of cancer live for ten years? I appreciate you could be that unlucky 1 per cent – but then any of us could also be knocked over by a bus or eaten by a lion (not so likely), or die in a plane crash (even less likely – unless you were on my flight a few years ago that included a loss of cabin pressure, the masks and lots of panic!).

I've always been scared of flying. We are not just talking a little jittery, we are talking full-on, bolt it to the front of the plane during take-off, screaming 'Let me off,' before being rugby-tackled to the ground by cabin crew kind of scared. The panic sets in a few days before a flight, when my body goes into adrenaline overdrive and I start researching all recent plane crashes and the safety records of my chosen airline. I reach new heights of 'embarrassing mum' status when I start knocking back the whisky at 6am at the airport and have a little snooze on a bench so that my name is boomed out on the tannoy to get my arse quickly to the gate, where I'm looked up and down by cabin staff who start debating if I'm in a fit state to fly. As I step onto a plane, the irrational side of me says that this is the most dangerous thing I can do – I'm going to die. Statistics, however, will tell you that even quantifying the risk of death from a plane crash is so minimal that a figure can't universally be agreed upon; but current argument falls at around one in 11 million. In fact you are more likely to die from the plane food itself (at a risk of one in 3 million), and if your plane does go down – well, a recent study found that 95.7 per cent of passengers will survive a crash.

So if, like me, you're scared even by these really quite good odds, how then do you deal with statistics that tell you you have more of a chance of dying in the next year than of surviving, and that the idea of living long enough to see your children make it to secondary school is now a distant pipe dream that needs parking in la-la land? That wasn't my plan for my life!

I had what some might call a rapidly accelerated journey through the cancer stages, and with each advancement (as is the case for nearly all cancer types), my chances of surviving for five years plummeted dramatically. From what looked like a benign tumour when first diagnosed, I went quickly to what turned out to be stage four cancer, with seven tumours in my lungs.

'So that means I only ever had an eight per cent chance of living!' I remember shouting at my surgeon, having read way too much about stage-four bowel cancer statistics. Then I bolted it straight to the local bar with my friend, where I sobbed into a whisky glass, planning my funeral. I was being faced with statistics that said I will not see my kids grow up, numbers that were telling me I didn't have a future; so I tried really hard to search for something that told me otherwise. I delved into parts of Google I never knew existed and found new search skills that even Bill Gates would have been impressed by. But the more I hunted the worse the picture got. I started to break my research down by age, location of tumour, tumour type, treatment plan etc. I even started studying oncology textbooks to understand the genetic make-up of the type of tumour I had and response percentages from various chemo trials. But every avenue I came across delivered more bad news for me. Not only did my research confirm that even with my plan of action my statistics were still appalling, I could find no positive factors that might help give me a boost. Instead, I had the worst of the worst: a tumour make-up that according to every research trial was the one you don't want, the one that has the lowest response to chemo and the shortest average survival time.

Now, your stats may paint a positive picture of hope – and I really hope they do – but if they don't, please do not lose hope. Learn that all the research in the world can't say exactly what will happen to YOU. Park it.

Recognise that continuing to study the stats will get you nowhere, apart from feeding a negative loop of anxiety. Accept that you will be a statistic, a little dot that others in the future might study. But neither you nor me, nor our healthcare teams, know which one dot you'll be, so for today learn to just live.

Some key things to consider doing when it comes to knowing your stats:

- Ask yourself – do you really want to know? What are you going to do with the result anyway?

- If you do look, only look at reputable sites (see opposite).
- Remember, your cancer is unique to you – and no research or even oncologist can totally predict how it will behave in your body.
- Statistics are based on older methods and regimes – think about new procedures developed in even the last few years. Their impact will take years to show up in statistics.
- Ask your oncologist for their opinion first.
- People will tell you not to look at statistics, but do whatever feels right for you...
- ... but don't keep looking at them. Know what you face and then park it. Nothing you will find will make them better.
- Do research trials, drug options and novel treatments – but check their validity. Who funded the research, what's the context, where are the results published?
- Ensure that you break down statistics, if they're available, by key sub-criteria such as stage type, age range, with/without chemo.
- Know that statistics don't tell *your* story.
- Know that statistics are all outdated and you are part of the ones to be published in five years' time.
- As hard as they may find them to read, refer family and friends to them – it can help contextualise your cancer and the reality of what you face.

If you want to do research into your cancer statistics, there are two sites I highly recommend. I'd suggest sticking to these (unless your oncologist recommends otherwise), and also just having a quick look and then try not to do it again! The information won't change and you must remember, stats are not you and YOUR cancer.

www.cancerresearchuk.org Here you can search by cancer type and stage. There is a wealth of approved statistics for the UK for all cancers.

www.mskcc.org/nomograms This is the New York-based Memorial Sloan Kettering Cancer Center website. It has an excellent predictor tool for survival and overall outcomes known as a prognostic nomogram. It is widely used by oncologists all over the world and, although it's free and easily accessible, I'd recommend only using it armed with medical knowledge gained from your oncologist as it doesn't cover all cancers and you will need some key medical information to complete it. Please think really carefully before using it, whether you really want to know that figure.

I've Become a Pincushion (Scans and Tests)

If you could always know what, medically, was going on inside your body, would you want to know? Would you want to know if you had weeks, months or a year to live – so you could work towards that day with looming fear? As a cancer patient you have to accept that tests and waiting for test results becomes an integrated part of your life and will determine your treatment plan. Each time you will wait with nervous anticipation of what might be and ride the emotional rollercoaster in the hope that the results will be kind.

Before cancer – or in my life BC, as I now call it – having a blood test was a big deal in my life. A referral from the GP, even for just a standard blood count, would send me over the edge. I'd nervously drive to my local hospital and wait, twiddling my thumbs and working myself up until I was called in. During the test I'd go weak in the head, thinking I was going to pass out – I'd look away and bite my lip in the hope that it would be over quickly. I'd then wobble back to the car eating a Mars Bar and drinking something sugary, believing that I'd just been through a massive ordeal and now needed a full day of resting and being pampered to recover. And yet now having blood tests, whether I like them or not, is as much a regular part of my life as working out.

Scan Anxiety Is Officially a Head-screw

Life with cancer is really 'life between scans'. You may well find yourself praying for a window of stability where the anxiety about what might be can take a back seat, at least until the next scan is upon you.

If you get claustrophobic when you have CT, PET or MRI scans you can, for at least parts of the procedure, ask to have someone in the room with you for distraction. While on the CT scanner I often recite positive thoughts out loud, sometimes to the alarm of the radiographers, who I forget can hear everything! Just remember that scans are an important part of monitoring your cancer and they help the healthcare team to determine the best plan of action. Think of them as helping you rather than as something to worry about.

There is, unfortunately, no alternative; however, there are some things you can do to help navigate scans and the results game better:

- If you really struggle with claustrophobia you can ask for some relaxation medication while you are being scanned.
- Tell the radiographers if you feel nervous. They can show you the room beforehand and talk you through what will happen.

- Just remember that the radiographers can hear you in the room. You can request they chat with you and give you a countdown of the time remaining.
- Jam-pack your diary while you're waiting for test results.
- Know that everyone worries about this.
- Always hope for the best rather than assuming the worst will happen – think positively.
- Don't be disappointed by a bad result – there are often lots of options (even at stage four).
- Push and chase to get results quickly. Ask wherever possible for a quick turnaround and a follow-up appointment asap. Sometimes I have even managed to get them the same day.

Doctor Relationships

When I first met my surgeon he told me straight away that I didn't have to choose him, but that if I did he promised to treat me like a daughter – and without a doubt he treated me brilliantly. You have to trust the team that support you – they are after all in charge of saving your life! When we discovered that my cancer was stage four, my oncologist promised me that he would do everything humanly possible to keep me alive – kitchen sink and all. Now that's the kind of thing you want to hear when faced with such uncertainty, so many questions and fear over just what the future holds.

Second Opinions

Many people assume that they are not entitled to change their healthcare team. I'm not going to say it's easy, and you will need to get a referral letter from either your GP or your existing team, but if you are not happy then do ask. I've known many people who have changed their entire team and hospital care because they were not happy with the set-up. Key points to remember when it comes to the patient/doctor relationship:

- Don't be afraid to ask questions – your healthcare team will always do their best to answer your concerns.
- You can question their options and choice of treatment for you even though they are highly regarded specialists.
- Remember it's your body and ultimately YOU are in control of YOUR care. You can choose to have treatment or not – it must be a two-way relationship.
- Be very open with your team about how you feel. You don't have to just nod politely. Voice your concerns and share your feelings.

Plans, Scans, Dots and Docs!

TAKE-AWAY TOP TIPS

Here are the take-away nuggets from this chapter to help you navigate from diagnosis to stats to docs:

Tip 1 Have an initial plan and know it may change – accept that this is part of living with cancer.

Tip 2 Think carefully about whether you want to look at statistics, and then park what you have found – they cannot say what will happen to you personally.

Tip 3 For statistics and prognosis, only look at reputable websites, and speak and listen first and foremost to your team.

Tip 4 Prepare for scans and know that they are there to help you – they are not the enemy; cancer is!

Tip 5 The relationship with your healthcare team is a two-way process – you need to trust them but also feel comfortable enough to question them. Get a second opinion if you are not happy.

• • •

'The good physician treats the disease: The great physician treats the patient who has the disease.'

William Osler

Chapter 4

Chemo Farts and Other Unexpected Side Effects

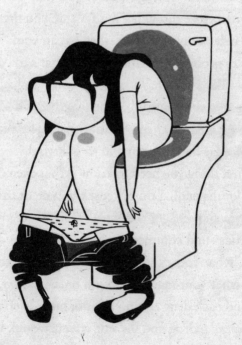

So you've been told you are having chemotherapy or possibly immunotherapy as a course of treatment. You have most likely heard horror stories and seen images of grey-looking patients and puke buckets – and yes, I'm going to be straight with you and tell you it happens. You may be in for a rough ride or you may be surprised at how you breeze through – but I assure you that if a girl with a needle phobia can do it, then so can you!

You are probably petrified about what's to come and you may, like I did, have no idea what a chemo cycle even was (for the record, it's the length of time it takes for one treatment of chemo to take place), let alone what one involved. I had to learn and so will you!

The first thing you need to know is that chemotherapy varies a lot depending on not just the type of cancer but also the stage of cancer you have. While there are standard practices and common regimes, be prepared for the fact that what you experience might not be exactly the same as what your mate, also with breast cancer, experiences. And each drug combo has unique side effects; just to explain each drug and the side effects would, I'm sure, take enough books to fill a small library! You will be given specific information on your likely side effects by your chemo nurse, but I have found www.macmillan.org. uk to be a wealth of easy-to-read information about most of the common chemo combinations, and it will at least provide you with a starting point.

So I'm 21 cycles and three regimes down (regimes being plans of action and different types of drugs that, in my case anyway, kept changing), have had more side effects than you could shake a stick at and am still sat here writing – albeit with tingling fingers! So let me share my tips to get you through.

Straight Down the Line (Ports, Lines and Needles)

'I'm not having another operation!' I screamed upon first meeting my oncologist. He had just told me that I'd be having a port fitted, which in my case would involve yet another general anaesthetic and yet more scars. 'Can't I just swallow a tablet?' I innocently asked, 'Or can't you just shove a needle in me each time?'

The first challenge, one that hadn't even entered my head pre-cancer, is getting the drugs into you. These are cytotoxic drugs that can, in some cases, cause burning when they go into smaller veins and even cause them to collapse. Yes, some chemotherapy is available in tablet form, but the majority is administered through intravenous drips directly into your veins. Depending on your regime, how long it is and, in some cases, on individual hospital practice, you may be fitted with either a port, a PICC line or a Hickman line. Here are some very helpful sources of information if you want to find out more:

Port	www.macmillan.org.uk/information-and-support/treating/chemotherapy/being-treated-with-chemotherapy/implantable-ports.html
PICC Line	www.macmillan.org.uk/information-and-support/treating/chemotherapy/being-treated-with-chemotherapy/picc-lines.html
Hickman Line	www.macmillan.org.uk/information-and-support/treating/chemotherapy/being-treated-with-chemotherapy/central-lines.html

Having protested like a child over getting my port fitted, I'm now grateful for this literal lifeline that has saved my veins – I proudly show it off as yet another 'war wound'. And, as well as it allowing me to just get on with my daily life, I have to admit to occasionally using it to get through airport security a little faster!

Needles

You are going to have to get used to them. During treatment you will have a lot – and I mean hundreds – of blood tests. They will be used to check everything from the functioning of your immune system to your liver and kidney functions to (for some cancers) specialised tumour marker tests. Again, these tests will be specific to your cancer, but rest assured that they will happen! Operations and the administration of some drugs require cannulas – oh and, just for laughs, you may even have a regime that requires you to inject yourself with an immune-boosting drug or hormones... and yes, for me the first time took an hour of leg-stabbing to get it in! So here are a few tips, from a needle-phobe, for how to get used to anything to do with needles:

- Ask for the numbing cream straight away.
- Lie down – it will stop you getting light-headed and ensure you don't sneak a peek at your arm and the needle.
- Look away.
- Breathe deeply and slowly. Keep calm as the needle goes in.
- Use the 'applied tension' technique – tense your large muscles to push your blood pressure up and stop yourself passing out.
- Visualise alternative scenarios – imagine you're lying on a beach!
- Gradually over time, and little by little, expose yourself to elements of the procedure.

Shaken Not Stirred (What Actually Happens at Chemo)

So you've turned up, nervous, not knowing what awaits you. Welcome to chemo club! Let's do this!

Your journey will start with you being told about all the side effects you can expect, how often you will have chemo, how many scans you'll have and when to expect them. I suggest taking your shoes off and ensuring that your phone is away and/or switched off; the first to ensure you don't go running out of the hospital, and the second to stop you googling every horror story around. But just remember that most people who have chemo cope pretty well on it. As long as you have the right healthcare team at your side, cheering you along, and helping you navigate through the bumps – you can do this.

It's important to note that many regimes and treatments now include a type of immunotherapy, either on its own or alongside chemotherapy. The process of many of these newer treatments is similar to chemotherapy, and the side effects, while for some people they might be reduced, may for others be on a par with chemo.

The actual process of having chemo or immunotherapy is different for everyone but some of the things you can expect are:

Pre-Assessment	Before you can have chemo, the doctors will need to ensure that your body is in a fit enough condition to handle it. They will run a battery of blood tests to check for different functions and to ensure that your immune system is working. Normally you will meet with a nurse or doctor to discuss the previous cycle and raise any concerns that you had about it. Chemo will then be given the go-ahead (or possibly not). **Present your symptom diary — be honest.**
Access and observations	This will involve either a nurse gaining access into your port or PICC line or, if you are getting the chemo through a cannula, inserting one. Refer to the tips on page 55. Normally your blood pressure, temperature and weight will be recorded. It's like Weight Watchers in reverse — weight gain or stabilisation is normally celebrated. **Breathe! Calm yourself as much as possible and know you can do this.**
Pre-Meds	Don't be alarmed! You will be given a plethora of medication beforehand to pre-empt reactions to your chemo drugs. This might include steroids, anti-sickness, antihistamine or anti-spasm drugs, to name but a few. Your nurses will then wait for these to take effect before administering the chemotherapy. Don't be alarmed if some of these drugs either hype you up or send you to a happy place of sleep and relaxation. If you need an extra bit of help — **ask for the magic blue pill! — a form of anti-anxiety medication that will help you relax.**

Cold Cap	For some regimes you may be offered the use of a cold cap to reduce hair loss. This will involve wetting and shampooing your hair and fitting an ice-cold cap as tightly to your scalp as possible. You will cry and you may decide it's not worth it; or you may just want to at least give it a shot and, like me, muddle your way through it. Remember not all chemo makes you lose your hair, and some regimes do not recommend the cold cap. Ask your healthcare team. **Distraction, distraction, distraction! Try a variety of techniques to get you through the first ten minutes and before you know it, you'll be a pro.**
Chemotherapy or immunotherapy drugs	You won't feel it going in. There may be one, two, three or even more drugs and they may be a combination of immunotherapy and chemotherapy drugs. They will come in a strict order and vary in how long they take to administer: some will take ten minutes; other will take hours and you may need to be admitted for an overnight stay. With some — like mine — you may leave the hospital while still attached to a portable chemotherapy pump that you can even take to the pub with you! The nurses will monitor you throughout for any signs of a reaction and continue with observations such as blood pressure. They are there ready to deal with any issues that might crop up. So if you are NOT feeling okay, just tell them. **Don't sit there waiting for an allergic reaction to the drugs. It might never happen!**

Post-chemotherapy drugs to manage side effects	Clear a space in your cupboards – you are setting up an at-home pharmacy! You will come home with bags of essential drugs and 'just-in-case' drugs and drugs you never knew existed! It's highly likely you will be given steroids and anti-sickness drugs at least for the first few days of each of your chemo cycles, to help your body manage the side effects. There has been a lot of research into the best combinations, so do take them, but if they don't work – let someone know! **Set alarms on your phone for when you should take the tablets each day – it will help you get into a routine.**

Ask Questions and Get Organised

The unknown is scary. The more I knew and understood about what would happen in my chemo regime, the more relaxed I felt. So ask questions and write things down. Ask for the names of your drugs so you can go away and look them up should you so wish. Your nurses will be only too happy to explain what is going in you and why. Write down the telephone numbers and contact details of any key hospital access points you are given; they're important. Ask for a print-off of your blood results each week and keep track yourself of how your body is coping each cycle.

My Biggest Fear

Nobody knows how they are going to react when they are given certain drugs. I have a history of allergic reactions ranging from strawberries to Aspirin. So it was just my luck that I was going to have allergic reaction to chemotherapy... Three so far, all of which have required lots of hydrocortisone and Piriton. The first time, as soon as the drugs went in it felt like I was having a massive panic attack, my heart started racing and my blood pressure was all over the place. The scariest one was on a new drug regime; I lost my ability to speak! Imagine going from zero to ten gin and tonics in a split second and slurring like an alcoholic wreck, but without the fun... There were lots of steroids and hand-holding and, while I was still slurring, at least over a few cycles, I regained my ability to speak and could continue the treatment.

It sounds, and was, frightening, but it also made me realise that the nurses are trained to be on guard and know what to watch for; at the press of a button nurses will come running and all will be fine. Seriously dangerous allergic reactions are actually quite rare, and in any case your team are highly skilled in dealing with them. I've lived to tell the tale of my adverse reactions, and you will too.

Call the Hotline!

In most hospitals you will be given a hotline number to call if you have any concerns while at home between treatment sessions. The doctors and nurses will be only too happy to provide answers to your questions, which can provide great comfort. Always remember: no question is too silly, you are not wasting anyone's time and you must put your health concerns first.

Get Into a Routine

Are you an organised person? How good are you at remembering to take your medication each day at the correct time? I struggle, but if you get into a routine it does make it a lot easier. Setting alarms on your phone each day is a great way of ensuring you take your tablets – and get a pillbox! Yes, they might remind you of your grandma, but it is quite satisfying dividing your tablets into each day!

Speak to Your Chemo Buddies

Most chemo wards are open chairs where (depending very much on your set-up) possibly 20 people will be having chemo all at the same time. People will make it clear if they fancy a chat or not. So, if you are up to it, talk to those who are up for it – you are in it together after all! And you will probably find you all share the same fears. It's not only nice to hear other people's stories; you may also pick up some excellent tips or golden nuggets of advice. The distraction of having a chat may make the hours pass more quickly.

I have met a few people on my ward who I still just love bumping into – even if it's partly just to affirm that we are all still kicking around. John has been going to the Marsden for 20 years and has seen it all; it gives me hope that if he's still around years after being told he had six weeks to live then I may well be too! Patrick makes me laugh, not least because we shared the same rather rare chemo reaction of losing our ability to speak. He too is a long-timer and has had cancer appear, disappear and reappear on numerous occasions but is still hopeful.

Take Backup (If You Feel Like It)

Do you take people with you to chemo or not? Choosing the right person is essential, and while people may kindly volunteer, don't feel it rude if you just want to say 'No, but thank you,' without explanation. Some days you will feel like only a good old girly natter with a friend will help calm the situation; other days you may want to be left alone. Even the most outwardly sociable of us (moi!) can on occasion just want to scuttle into it, do it alone and scuttle on home. Be honest with your friends – if you feel sick and don't want to chat, then really don't feel you need to.

It's Not a Place For Children…

I was hooked up to a chemo pump about to start my 15th cycle when I got a phone call from my daughter's school to say she had got a ring stuck on her finger and needed taking to hospital to cut it off. You couldn't make this up! With everyone else who'd normally be able to help not available, I jumped into the car to the school, to be met with a laughing eight-year-old who was enjoying being the centre of attention. Yes, she needed the ring off, but it could wait; I knew that if I didn't return to the hospital in time I'd be refused chemo for the day as there simply wouldn't be time to administer it. So I decided to take her back to the chemo ward with me.

For the last ten months she'd been asking, with childhood curiosity, just what happened when I had chemo, and I knew she worried about Mummy. Her little road trip enabled her to see first-hand what it was actually like, to debunk the imaginings and nightmares that her little mind might have been creating; and she had fun riding on the chemo pumps. A few packs of crisps and an iPad kept her occupied and from that moment on she stopped being worried when I said 'I'm having chemo.' I wouldn't advocate it on a first run, but if your children are old enough and are asking, show them! It's not as scary as their little minds might think.

Dress For the Occasion

On some cycles you may want to turn up in your most comfortable tracksuit, hand-warmers in bag and big scarf to hide in from the world. Other times, if you want to don a pair of Louboutins, a miniskirt and bright red lipstick, then do it. Whatever you feel like doing is perfectly acceptable as long as you can access the treatment. The nurses will be only too happy to take pictures.

I've Got This – Oh No, No I Don't!

The effects of chemo are, on the whole, cumulative, but don't be surprised if you feel surprisingly well during the first few cycles. And for some people for most of the treatment. For me the effects crept up on me until, wham, I felt like I'd hit a brick wall – it was in cycle 18 and it made me realise that it was starting to have a massive impact on my daily life. My neuropathy – loss of sensation in my hands and feet – was totally manageable until

I woke up one morning and felt like I'd aged 50 years. Talk honestly to your team about any side effects you are experiencing and they can help you.

What's Normal?!

You will discover a new normal and realise that anything is possible at any time. If you are on chemo for a long time, you may begin to recognise a pattern of symptoms so you can plan your days accordingly. However, don't be surprised, or down on yourself, if you make a plan, thinking you're going to have a good day, and instead you can't get out of bed. Just be kind to yourself and say you'll plan for another good day instead.

Your Cycles

This might be once a week, once every two weeks or longer depending on your cancer. You may like to plan the cycles out in a calendar so you can start ticking off each one – be proud when you've completed one and make sure you reward yourself! It can also be useful to visualise and map out (after a few cycles) what an average cycle looks like for you. This might help you plan some really nice things to do on your 'good days' and to know in advance when you'll need those duvet days. For me, while it always varied a little, over time it became more predictable, and yours might too. This is what my average cycle looked like:

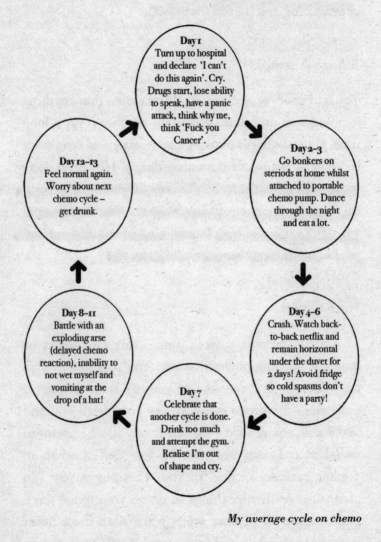

Day 1
Turn up to hospital and declare 'I can't do this again'. Cry. Drugs start, lose ability to speak, have a panic attack, think why me, think 'Fuck you Cancer'.

Day 2-3
Go bonkers on steriods at home whilst attached to portable chemo pump. Dance through the night and eat a lot.

Day 4-6
Crash. Watch back-to-back netflix and remain horizontal under the duvet for 2 days! Avoid fridge so cold spasms don't have a party!

Day 7
Celebrate that another cycle is done. Drink too much and attempt the gym. Realise I'm out of shape and cry.

Day 8-11
Battle with an exploding arse (delayed chemo reaction), inability to not wet myself and vomiting at the drop of a hat!

Day 12-13
Feel normal again. Worry about next chemo cycle – get drunk.

My average cycle on chemo

When Things Don't Go According to Plan

Sometimes You May Need a Strong Mate to Drag You to Your Chemo Chair

I had some 'unusual' reactions to chemotherapy. And as a result I got scared. To the point that it would take two nurses and lots of talking to myself to convince me that I could go through with the next cycle. You may have days where you are kicking and screaming (at least inside), all inner 'fight' has left en route to hospital and you don't really know where you will find the mental capacity to go through with it – but you will. It will take support, it will take some firm words with yourself and it will take every ounce of strength you never knew you had. I found that mapping out my thought process (see my example overleaf) helped me turn those negative thoughts into a more positive mindset. Why not get yourself a journal and try mapping your thoughts so you too can 'catch' your negative process and flip it.

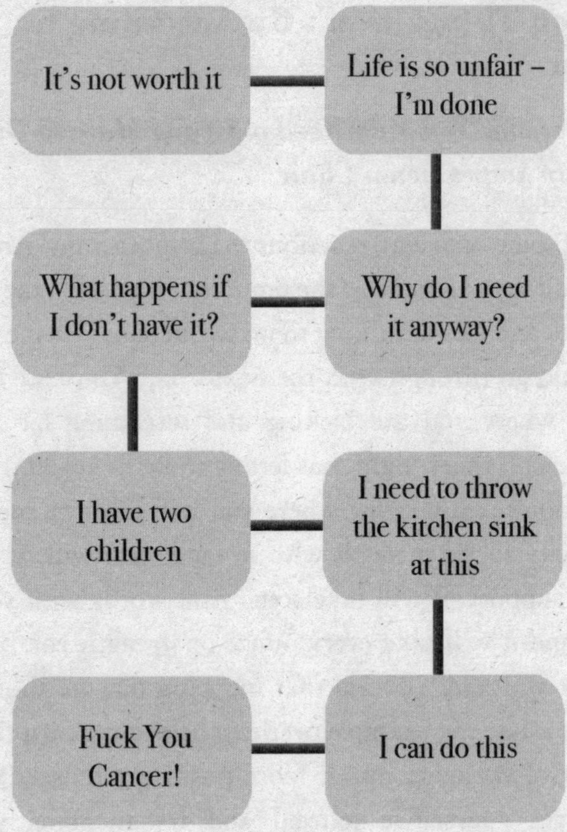

My thought process before chemo

Treat Yourself

One strategy to get through it to reward yourself at the end of each cycle – it's the little things! Ideally of course we'd all be buying ourselves an expensive pair of shoes, a handbag or an Aston Martin each time... but back in the real world – try out some of these ideas:

Buy a new fragrance and wear it to each chemo cycle.	Plan a cinema trip/ night out after a cycle.	Wine and cheese night.
A new pair of PJs or an item of comfy clothing.	Some new underwear.	A new book.
An afternoon in front of the telly – an old black-and-white film or your daytime-TV guilty pleasure.	Catch up with an old friend you haven't seen in a while.	Write a letter to your future self reminding yourself how awesome you are!
Have one day of 'me time' to look forward to – bath, candles, a good night's sleep.	Raise your sock game! Get yourself a new pair each time.	Treat yourself to a new plant for the garden.

When Chemo is Suspended

Your doctors may well suspend your chemotherapy. This can happen for a variety of reasons: a change in treatment, a body that doesn't want to play ball or just because it's half-term. Don't be surprised if you plan to have a non-chemo week but suddenly it becomes a chemo week and that spa weekend or National Trust visit you were looking forward to is when you will now be vomiting. You will feel frustrated – but when your chemo is suspended, if you can, make the most of it (think of it as a mini free pass!). Don't forget to get some rest and eat well to get you back on track.

Make It Work For You Too

You are living through this treatment. This is your reality, and while your health is the number one thing to focus on in your life right now, you also need reasons to live, things to look forward to and a break from the treatment cycle. If it's medically safe to do so and you want to take a holiday, then be vocal about that. Or perhaps you have a special day coming up – a wedding, a party – and being hooked up to a chemo pump will ruin the outfit you've been planning for six months! Let your team know and they will bend over backwards to make it work for you.

When the BIG Plan Changes

Chemo doesn't always work to shrink or halt tumour growth. That is the harsh reality of these clever little nuclear beasts. I was told to expect 12 cycles, but 21 cycles later, I was still going – and who knows what the future holds. I joke now that I may be on chemo for life – but it's not entirely a joke; I could be. If your cancer grows while you're on chemo, your regime may be classified as failing or as you having had no response. We all dream about a total pathological response whereby the tumours are zapped by the drugs and we go on our merry way. I started getting depressed by scans that showed stability – in other words, no change – but now, as a stage-four patient, I jump for joy at stable scans, knowing that they could fall off a cliff at any moment. I'm on my third regime, and as each has passed I start to worry that my options are running out.

If you are told your chemo has failed it's totally normal to:

- Feel cheated, as though you've run a marathon and someone has moved the finish line.
- Feel a sense of losing faith in your body's ability to tackle this.
- Wonder if your healthcare team are right for the job and question everything they've done to date.
- Feel a loss of hope and maybe that it's game over.

But as they say – without sounding totally morbid – it's not over until it's really over! Stay hopeful, challenge

F*** YOU CANCER

your team, hunt for options and get second, third and fourth opinions.

When Drugs Are Not Available on the NHS

The NHS is incredible – but you may find yourself in a situation where a type of treatment is only available to you privately. If you have been told there is nothing more that can be done, go back to your oncologist and ask a philosophical question – if money was no object what could be done? If there are options, start researching. Find out how you can gain access, what's the likelihood it will work for you, what are the side effects. Swallow your pride and crowdfund. People are on the whole very happy to provide financial support if you can explain what kind of treatment you are having and why and that it's not some wild, unproven, crazy regime at a dodgy clinic at the end of a rough dirt track! For more information on crowdfunding check out www.crowdcube.com.

Trials

Research holds the key to living with cancer but at what point, if at all, are you prepared to be the guinea pig? I think trials offer an opportunity not only to prolong your life, but also to pave for the way for future

72

generations. Be aware that there are strict criteria for all trials and you will need to work closely with your oncologist to explore what options are available to you. For a list of trials currently recruiting check out www.cancer-researchuk.org/about-cancer/find-a-clinical-trial.

Chemo Brain

Every day I lose something. It's normally my keys and then my phone – and then I find my phone and realise the keys are lost again. It can sometimes take an entire episode of *Jeremy Kyle* for me to realise my keys are, in fact, in front of me and my phone is in my pocket. And this, ladies and gentlemen, is called chemo brain. While chemotherapy was nuking all those cancer cells it was also screwing up your brain – surprise! No one really tells you about this until afterwards, probably in the hope that by the time you recognise you have chemo brain, your memory will forget that you do! My first warning signs were when I started struggling to follow conversations at a party. I felt like my brain was working overtime to keep up and I came home exhausted.

Be prepared for a memory like a goldfish – which is a great excuse for forgetting birthdays – concentration like a child with ADHD and a multitasking ability that leaves the term juggling firmly in the circus ring! You will need to give yourself more time to do 'life admin' and all the boring shit that – if you are anything like me – you hate doing anyway. Try to outsource where you can – if you can afford to, maybe get a cleaner, or pay someone to iron your shirts – but recognise that even the best of us need to pay our own parking fines when the cancer card has well and truly failed!

Added Extras!

My biggest advice to you is don't suffer in silence. Unless you are Superman you will have side effects. These can range from feeling sick to hair loss, a plummeting immune system and just about everything in between – including some weird ones. For me this included an inability to be out in cold weather without my hands and mouth moving on their own accord! I suggest that you understand what to expect and don't focus on these symptoms too much. It's unique for everyone and if you start to overthink it, a few new ones might even creep in. But you do need to keep track of what happens to you and to understand what is expected and when to call your nurse. There are amazing drugs, for example, to counteract sickness and many other side effects, but they don't always get it right first time. So if you are taking anti-sickness tablets and you still feel sick, ask for alternatives. Why not:

- Use a cancer notebook/journal (with a nice cover to distract you from what's inside) to record all your side effects in one place. Take this with you to each appointment.
- Rank or rate your side effects – perhaps on a 1–5 scale, with 5 being totally incapacitating and 1 being a mild annoyance.
- Ask a friend or relative to read your list of side effects. Get them to be your first point of contact. That way you can run worries through them before the doctors.
- As always, if you are ever unsure of anything – call your team.

Your New Skills

We all fart. Some are loud and proud, some smelly and silent – but we are all capable of producing a bubbly concoction from our backsides. Now prepare yourself – and by prepare I mean, get yourself a nose peg, buy a dog and warn everyone who lives with you that due to chemotherapy your stomach is about to change – and not for the better. You will discover a new-found ability to produce a stench you thought was only possible for a year's worth of decomposing cabbage. The dog is needed so that you have someone else to blame the smell on when your in-laws are over for dinner.

There will be those moments when you laugh because otherwise you'll cry – but at the time you will not find it funny. It is, in fact, possible to vomit, poo, wee, cry and have a nosebleed all at the same time, and the only question you'll be asking is which end do you point towards the toilet. Hell, if we lived in a society that valued bodily functions as the gold standard, you'd be the star of the show!

My most interesting side effect while I was on chemotherapy – while I didn't find it at all funny at the time, in retrospect I can laugh about it – was the one where my hands moved involuntarily. They actually spasmed while the chemo drugs were pumped in and whenever I got cold. I wore oven gloves to open the fridge and a hot-water bottle became my new best friend. And if I took a walk down my local high street in the middle of winter when I was on oxaliplatin (a bowel cancer drug), I had to be prepared for serious facial spasms that looked like I had been taking drugs of a whole different kind!

Your body will produce sounds, movements and reactions you never thought humanly possible and

I suggest you laugh whenever you can – otherwise you will just cry!

Keep a Symptom Diary

To become accustomed to your new-found talents you may find it useful, at least at the beginning, to keep a diary. This can be as simple as just a few notes each day in your cancer journal, or as complex as a rating spreadsheet. Whatever you use, your diary will help to ensure that you discuss fully with your team everything you are experiencing, and so will help you to get the right medication to control the symptoms. For each symptom ask: *Is this intolerable, or just a nuisance? Is it affecting my quality of life?*

You may find a table like the one below useful; it's easy to follow and will give you an overview of your cycle progress:

Day	Sickness	Tiredness	Hair loss	Skin	Bowel	Neuropathy	Other
1	None	Normal	-	-	Constipation	Hands cold in fridge	Itching
2	None	Lots of energy	Thinned on brushing	Red cheeks	Back to normal	Spasm after cold	-

My Diary Extracts

> **21 April 2016:** 'Fucker of a day. No energy. Watched 10 episodes of *Friends*. Vomit x 3. Poo x 6. Arms and legs feel heavy. Scar from operation is hurting but paracetamol worked. 2 naps.'
>
> **24 April 2016:** 'Good day – got drunk.'
>
> **25 April 2016:** 'Bollocks I'm hungover. Now I feel sick again. Poo x 8. Imodium taken. Headache. Is this self-inflicted or chemo?!'

Expect the Unexpected

While for some people the cycles may be predictable, expect the unexpected. After 18 cycles my stomach decided to start exploding (imagine norovirus and then some), having never really done so before, and suddenly in cycle 12 my heart went nuts! But a few tests later and all was okay. Be alert and aware of your body and know what is normal for you. Report anything you have concerns over. Even if it means an extra day in hospital, it will be much easier to sleep in the knowledge that you've been checked out rather than worry over what might be.

Be Kind to Yourself

Chemo is physically and mentally tiring. Your body is going to go through a lot and you will at times wonder how that head is coming off the pillow without a Red Bull. You will have days when you just want to sleep, days when you just want to eat and days when you just want to run into a hole and never reappear. At 3am when you have vomited your entire stomach contents onto the floor for the fifth time that day, you will say 'I can't do this.' But learn to be kind to yourself. Learn that you will have good days and bad days – and some very bad days (or you may not). But give yourself a break. Tomorrow is another day, and that just might be a great one!

Did You Wash Your Hands?

I give you permission to be anal over hygiene and illness. In fact you need to be. You will have the immune system of a baby (if you are lucky) and there will be days of your cycle when coming into contact with anyone who is ill can be extremely dangerous. Chemo has the potential to wipe out an aspect of your immune system called neutrophils, which help your body fight infection. Simply put, no neutrophils = neutropenia = life-threatening (if you come into contact with an infection) and you will be hot-footing it to hospital rather than enjoying a lazy round of Sunday golf! So, without locking yourself away and wrapping up in cotton wool, here are some simple things to do to help yourself stay germ-free:

- Buy a big bottle of hand sanitiser and stick it by your front door – ask everyone to use it.
- Tell people who are ill or who have ill children to stay away until they feel better.
- If you do need to travel, buy a mask from the chemist and use it – don't worry about what you look like.
- Become obsessive about washing your hands – get into a routine of doing it before every meal at least. Do you actually know how to wash your hands properly? It might sound like a simple thing to do, but the difference between doing it properly or not can be literally a life! Did you know that washing your hands properly should take the same amount of time as singing 'Happy Birthday'? Look up 'How to wash your hands' on the NHS website.

Radiotherapy

Just when you think it's only the nuclear drugs you need to navigate your way through, you may start a whole regime of radiotherapy. Not having had experience of radiotherapy myself, I've asked my friend Rhiannon Bradley to give you a little insight into what you might expect:

As someone who has battled with cancer twice, I've had my fair share of treatments. Between thyroid and breast cancer, I have had chemotherapy, surgery, radioactive iodine treatment and radio-therapy. Before cancer, if someone mentioned 'radi-otherapy' I would imagine lying in a big machine, lights down low, being zapped with radioactive laser beams, momentarily turning into some kind of glowing cancer superhero! Of course it wasn't quite as dramatic as this but, as with any cancer treat-ment, you don't really know what to anticipate until it happens to you.

I was given radiotherapy after chemotherapy and surgery to treat my breast cancer. Before my treat-ment began people told me it would be 'a walk in the park,' 'a breeze' and, the most popular response, 'a doddle compared to chemo.' 'Oh good,' I thought. As a busy mum of a toddler I decided to believe them and I was looking forward to a treatment that was going to be less emotionally and physically demanding.

As you can imagine, though, it wasn't quite the 'smooth ride' I had been expecting.

Before I started my radiotherapy, I was given a 'planning appointment' where I had some scans to determine where to position the machine that delivers the high-energy rays. This needs to be accurate as the radiographers need to ensure they only eradicate cancer cells. While I lay down, the team used rulers to measure me and draw dots in all the right places. Some of these were made permanent (like little tattoos) to make the treatment efficient and precise. They explained that due to the location of my tumour, I would need to hold my breath for up to 25 seconds during each treatment to lift my heart so it didn't get zapped by the rays. I was a bit worried about this as it seemed a long time to hold your breath!

I was keen to start as I had 20 treatments over the month of December. As the timing was pretty rubbish, I had decided that I wanted to make the whole experience more bearable by treating myself to something every time I had a session. I felt as though I deserved a little reward for all I'd been through. I decided that as I was preparing to go into battle mode, what could be better than a little bit of 'warpaint'? For every radiotherapy treatment I had, I treated myself to a new lipstick, which I documented on my Instagram blog @thebigcandme.

My first appointment was on a machine called LA 9 or Linear Accelerator. Lipstick applied, positive pants on, I arrived, removed my clothes from the waist up and lay down. As I lay there, arms above my head with everything on display, I must admit I felt self-conscious and exposed, but I soon realised that what they were interested in was inside my body, not outside! Once I was positioned correctly (to the millimetre), I was left alone. I listened to their instructions, held my breath when I needed to and before I knew it, it was all over. The whole event took roughly 20 minutes. Most of the time was spent getting me into position and the radiotherapy itself was painless, like having an X-ray.

As the weeks went by, I got into the swing of things. I built up a lovely rapport with the radiographers looking after me. I would try to make it fun and take in treats to keep us all going. My favourite memory is bringing in Santa hats for us to wear while we conducted my treatment to add a little festive cheer! However, as time passed, the process became harder. I was tired, my breast was getting increasingly painful and trying to organise child-care every day was a constant juggling act. I was tearful and often had a good cry in the car on the hour's car journey home from hospital. I had been mentally unprepared for how hard I would find it. I had expected this to be easy and painless; however it was definitely not the 'walk in the park' I'd been promised! The most challenging part for me was when it had all finished and my side effects were at their peak. My skin was frazzled and beginning to peel away from my breast and nipple. I had stabbing pains, fatigue and generally felt under the weather. However, after a few weeks I began to feel more myself as the pain subsided and my new skin emerged.

Throughout my treatment various people passed on their advice for helping with the side effects of radiotherapy such as staying hydrated, practising mindfulness to help me stay calm during treatments and keeping aloe vera gel in the fridge for extra comfort when I applied it to my damaged skin. Radiotherapy is not an 'easy' treatment but it gave this busy mum 20 minutes a day to lie down and an excuse to treat myself to a new lipstick – all the while curing me of breast cancer.

Chemo Farts and Other Unexpected Side Effects

TAKE-AWAY TOP TIPS

You've got this! Here are the take-away nuggets from this chapter to get you through chemo:

Tip 1 Understand your drugs and ask questions.

Tip 2 Keep a symptom diary.

Tip 3 Treat yourself during each cycle.

Tip 4 You can, and will, bounce back from a change of plan.

Tip 5 Appreciate and laugh at the new talents your body has!

Tip 6 Be kind to yourself and recognise you will have good and bad days.

Tip 7 Become anal about infection control (but don't lock yourself away!).

If all else fails, don a pair of heels or a sassy shirt and act as though you're nailing chemo as you strut onto the ward. It might just help – well, that or the Champagne you smuggled in with you!

• • •

'Give a girl the right shoes and she can conquer
the world.'

Marilyn Monroe

Chapter 5

Can Everyone Just Fuck Off? Support and Relationships

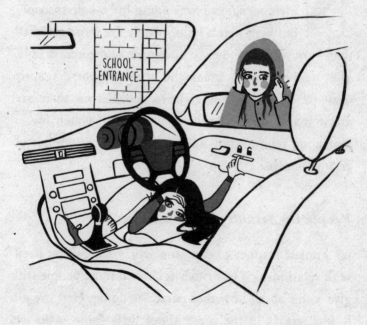

You Really DO Care, Don't You? (Telling People)

Now, I'm an extrovert by nature (I once told half my colleagues I was going for a colonoscopy) but I get that a lot of people are more reserved than I am when it comes to disclosure of medical details. How you choose to break the news of your diagnosis must sit with what feels right to you. For me there are a few main considerations and things to watch for in managing relationships in the immediate aftermath of your diagnosis:

People Do Actually Care How You Are

It's human instinct to care and worry for others. Even with relationships five times removed, most people still give a shit about how that person is doing. Hell, we all follow stories in the press about little Jonny who we don't know with incurable cancer, with nervous anticipation, desperately hoping it will all be okay in the end.

Online, people from all over the world, most of whom I've never met, follow me, and if I haven't posted anything for a while I get a barrage of messages essentially asking if I'm still alive! I'm always flattered – although explaining that I haven't posted simply due to having been eating McDonald's and watching TV for three days is less exciting than some medical emergency (God forbid). Like anyone would be, I was touched by each and every person who took the time to think of me when cancer first hit the fan. It got me through the really dark moments at the beginning to think that people were there walking with me. If you don't have someone to walk with you – remember there are lots of fabulous organisations listed in the back that will give you that much-needed helping hand.

No Joy in Repetition

So you've told your nearest and dearest what's happening. But then the next 'layer' of people want to know and friends of friends want to know and before you know it the postman is asking for a daily update and you fear the school gate for the new-found cancer celebrity status that you have been given. At first the attention is flattering and you willingly wax lyrical over a cuppa about the intimate details of your brand-new ability to shit out of your stomach. And then the questions start.

And sometimes you actually want to thump those who ask them.

What does stage four mean? What's your prognosis? What happens during chemo? How are you? And the most annoying – 'Are you really okay, honey?' (said in that patronising tone with the head tilt). In my mind my response goes along the lines of: 'Honestly, I'm crap. I'm surprised I'm holding it together today – I've spent the night coughing my guts into a bowl while simultaneously shitting into the toilet and stuffing my nose with loo roll to stop it bleeding.' Knowing full well that if that *were* to blurt out of my mouth, even the most unsqueamish person would flinch – and then respond with 'Oh darling what can I do to help?', in answer to which I wouldn't have the energy to think of anything. Therefore I tended to find it simpler to just say 'Oh I'm fine thanks'!

Repeating and explaining where you are in your treatment, what happens next and what that means may get to be just a little too much at times. Feel free to tell people that you just don't want to chat about it. It also helps to have one point of contact, a person who updates people with your treatment plan and how you are getting on – that way it's not you who's always the one fending off questions. Try blogging or setting up an email or text group – sometimes it's easier just to say things once and in one go.

Many people choose not to share their diagnosis, for a variety of reasons. If you choose this path, and whatever your reasons might be, make sure it's not just because you feel embarrassed by it. Cancer is nothing to be ashamed of – remember that one in two of us will receive a diagnosis in our lifetimes. I've had many people who have come forward and finally shared their cancer story, having been embarrassed by it for years. Those who hid it from everyone but their partner, carried on working as if nothing was going on and hid it from their little ones so as not to worry their young minds. For them, brushing it under the carpet was their coping mechanism and one just as valid as shouting it from the rooftops. You will know what feels right for you – but be aware that this may change over time and during your treatment. Just roll with it! Here are some key pointers for you to consider:

- Be as public or private as you want to be.
- Don't be embarrassed about or ashamed of your cancer.
- Don't feel that having cancer is a weakness.
- Accept the outpouring of well-wishes, love and support – it's the way others will deal with your diagnosis.
- Seek help from charities and look for support from those who have also experienced your cancer type and treatment.
- Give people hard facts.

- Don't feel bad if the advice people give you annoys you. It's inevitable that it sometimes will.
- Expect your relationships with just about EVERYONE to change – some for the good, some for the bad – everything is normal.
- You do not need to deal with or comfort those around you. Make yourself a priority – focus on your emotions and your treatment.
- People will have their own issues relating to cancer; expect some people to start acting strangely.

We All Need a Little Helping Hand!

I'm a headstrong, active 36-year-old who believes she can handle life (at times). Why on earth would I, of all people, need help, even while on chemo, to feed myself, walk my dog or generally put one foot in front of the other? If I can handle 1,500 teenagers on a daily basis, I can handle this... she thought! But cancer is a leveller like no other. A beast I underestimated. I have never felt so tired. So tearful, so scared, so alone and so sick – and yet I've never felt so loved and supported either.

I thought I could do this, and I can – and YOU CAN. But I never envisaged that there would be days when I struggled to lift my head off the pillow physically, or moments when I couldn't think straight for crying. It is because of the incredible people that I'm so blessed to have in my life (mum, dad, hubby, mates – I mean you!), that I'm able to function. As much as it pains me to feel like a pathetic child, I do need my hair to be held back while vomiting – and you just might need it too!

Although many people do, in my opinion cancer is not something to tackle alone. Build your army, build it strong and use it well. Now is the time in your life to swallow your pride, pull in those IOUs, ask for and accept all the help you can lay your hands on. You may think you want to do this alone, but I warn you – it's hard; and at some point, you may just want your hubby (or sadly, in my case, my 10-year-old son) to cuddle you at 3am and wipe away those tears – no matter how old you are. I appreciate that this is easily done if you are very lucky and are blessed with a fantastic family and friend network, but if you are on your own, ask your hospital about what help they can provide for you. I'm not advocating having someone around 24/7 – because there will be times when you want everyone just to go away – but it's always a nice surprise when I say I'm not hungry but an egg sandwich appears on the table in front of me anyway... and makes it nicely into my stomach. Now that's the kind of practical help I'm talking about! It brings tears of happiness to my eyes when I'm sat attached to a chemo pump in hospital and a mum friend sends me a text to say she's ordered an extra World Book Day costume for my daughter – THANK YOU! In an ideal world us cancer club members would all live in a 'Cancer Hotel' while we were undergoing treatment. We'd become best of buddies overnight, because let's face it, talking about our chemo side effects can keep us entertained for days! Five-star luxury on tap, meals that just turn up and a suspension of anything 'real world' to deal with. Of course there would be a shopping centre, yoga studio, gardening club, manicures and massages, a beach, fine dining and a theatre. Oh, and the endless woodland where you can just go and take a deep breath whenever you need to escape. You'd pop into the hospital section for your chemo, emerge to a bespoke recovery programme and recuperate for the next cycle while gazing in wonder at the sunset – and sipping margaritas of course! Oh, and naturally there'd be no bill at the end. While I'm still working on a business proposal to make this dream a reality, back in the real world we all need to find a way to orchestrate help to function and keep our daily lives ticking over so that things are not overbearing or tiring and you can just focus on riding through your cancer treatment. Even when the kids are screaming for lack of matching socks, or the CEO needs the report yesterday.

'Am I being a burden?' is a question that often comes to mind, as yet again my sister takes an afternoon off work to accompany me to chemotherapy. But help can come in a variety of shapes, and if you either don't feel or don't want to use those closest to you for whatever reason, there are lots of avenues you can explore. Each avenue may provide you with an element of unexpected support that can bring a glimmer of sunlight and laughter in even the darkest times.

There are lots of areas you may need help with – some obvious and some less so:

- Getting to and from hospital appointments – you may not be in the right state to drive yourself, or get on public transport.
- Managing the cancer admin – the relentless form-filling, waiting for phone calls, getting to speak to the right people and fighting your corner.
- Taking in the information presented – your mind may go numb in a hospital setting and therefore it's helpful to have someone to rely on to be able to repeat the conversation back to you at a later date.
- Financial support – do you have sick leave, will you still continue to work, how will you pay the mortgage?
- Ensuring you have the right medication on tap – or if you don't, having someone to run out to get it for you.

- Being forced to get out of bed – sometimes it takes a scheduled coffee with a friend to get you to function.

- Emotional support – who will you talk to about your darkest fears, the ones you find it the hardest to verbalise?

- A companion for operations, chemo, radiotherapy – spending lonely hours in hospital makes your mind dwell on the worst things.

- Someone to ensure you are fed properly – you may feel too weak to organise this yourself at points in your treatment. Never underestimate the power of food!

- Childcare – do you have a backup when you are stuck in hospital attached to a chemo pump and the school calls to say (for example …) your daughter got a ring stuck on her finger that needs cutting off?

- Dog care – yes, they are like having a newborn baby!

It's natural to turn at first to those nearest and dearest. Husband, wife, best friend. They will feel helpless at hearing your diagnosis, and as an innocent bystander will, in most cases, be desperately trying to make everything okay. But we all are only human at the end of the day; your nearest and dearest can absolutely provide solace, but even the most loving partner doesn't miraculously turn into the best carer or suddenly know exactly how you feel now you're having to face having cancer. There are lots of other places you can go to get targeted support.

Social Media

Up until my diagnosis I hadn't ever logged into Instagram and I didn't really know too much about blogging. I mean, I'd heard of it, but I had no understanding of the power and size of the network that lurked behind those little squares. I never imagined that engaging in these online 'worlds' would bring so many amazing people into my life – and, most importantly, people who could really support me emotionally and practically with what I was going through.

Engaging in the online world is not for everyone, and if it doesn't feel right to you – don't do it! However, if you do, and if you look carefully enough, you'll find a bank of inspirational people that might just perk you up in those low moments.

Charities and Cancer Support Centres

But I'm not a charity case, I used to think. I had charities all wrong. Until I got cancer I was naive about what they did and who they helped. When you are first diagnosed, you will google, and quite often Dr Google will present you with a barrage of information from charity websites. And you know what, this is the good stuff! It's verified, high-quality, well-researched information; if you are looking for the facts then charities' websites are the place to go. As well as invaluable information, you will find a community of support, of passionate people working very hard to really make a difference for people like you and me.

You may become attracted to charities for a variety of reasons. Perhaps you'll find the support and advice they can provide invaluable – in a lot of cases they have a wealth of experience, often with patients in similar situations, and they can therefore offer a great deal of comfort. For some it might be the research they fund to ensure no one else has to ride the cancer rollercoaster.

You or those close to you may well wish to fund-raise. This can help your nearest and dearest feel like they are doing something worthwhile and practical and it most certainly is welcome from charities' point of view! My advice to you is to research the organisations you may want to raise money for and ensure you have an understanding of how and where the money raised will go. What's their purpose, and what difference will your money make? I set up a team (Team Bowelbabe) on Just Giving and decided that all the money I'd raise would go to Bowel Cancer UK. I'd looked at how they use their money, and some of their research projects, like 'Never Too Young', really resonated with me. The charity's staff, including CEO Deborah Alsina, had also reached out to me from the moment I started mentioning the words 'bowel cancer' online and as such swept me up into their family of support. And I could not be more grateful.

Charity Fundraising

Bottom line: it's harder than you might think! I thought oh, I'll just raise loads of cash alongside doing my treatment – it will be easy. But I realised quickly that, while every little counts, boy do you need to sell a lot of cakes to make an impact! If you have the energy to throw a ball instead, or encourage people to sign up to a variety of running races, it will save you hours of slaving in the kitchen!

Charities are also always on the hunt for campaigners and case studies so that they can continue to raise funds to support others in your situation and to work on preventing others in the future having to face what you have. You will find they are passionate about creating this change.

One big subject is the taboos that still exist around issues such as women's health and – very close to my own heart – bowel health. One of the most high-profile organisations in this area is the Eve Appeal (see resources section), which is concerned with smashing the taboos around gynaecological health; but there are also many other charities who will be only too happy to welcome you in if you wish to support them in their missions to start and continue an open conversation about 'embarrassing' or taboo issues.

The Importance of Talking Taboos

Are you furious at your cancer? Do you think it's unfair that anyone has to go through the gruelling treatment you have to? Are you angry that you were diagnosed late, your symptoms weren't picked up or that awareness of your cancer is poor?

Often people experience symptoms but put off going to the GP, sometimes because they don't know what these symptoms might mean and sometimes because they find them embarrassing and don't want to talk about them. I mean, how many people do *you* know who can talk about poo with a straight face or without squirming?

But being able to talk openly about changes to bowel function, and all the other things that many of us find excruciatingly embarrassing, is vital.

As well as investigating charities' activities in this area, as discussed above, you could also work closer to home by encouraging those nearest and dearest to you to start talking openly about the things that make many of us uncomfortable; by doing so we could save lives.

Your hospital will be able to direct you towards charities specific to you, but here are a few more general places to start:

Cancer Research UK	www.cancerresearchuk.org
Maggie's Centres	www.maggiescentres.org
Macmillan	www.macmillan.org.uk
Shine Cancer Support	www.shinecancersupport.org
Look Good Feel Better	www.lookgoodfeelbetter.co.uk

It's wise to ensure the right support network is in place – for those around you as well as for yourself – and this can mean calling in reinforcements. We will talk more later about how partners and other family might deal with your illness, but for now I'll say that you are likely to be the first to notice the cracks; family members will all too often go into overdrive, believing that suddenly they can take on EVERYTHING and cope with the emotional rollercoaster at the same time. Direct them to the charities above for support – just as you will find them invaluable, so will they.

Please also have a look at the resources section at the back of this book for a fuller list of useful charity contact details.

Hospital Services

What, my hospital offers reflexology – for free?! I didn't know this! Hospitals offer a variety of free services to cancer patients – this will vary from hospital to hospital but can range from reflexology to massages to painting workshops, yoga and 'Look Good Feel Better' workshops. However, it's not always obvious that they exist; you do need to hunt down and proactively ask about the added extras. You will be allocated a clinical nurse specialist who will oversee your treatment – they will be able to point you in the right direction. Make the most of it. I attended one of the workshops mentioned above (and see Chapter 7 for more information). I was apprehensive about going – I don't need to be just 'cancer' all the time, I thought to myself. But what I found surprised me. A great bunch of women, sharing their stories, having a laugh in the trenches together – it was wonderful. So try it out – you too might be surprised!

I Love You More Today Than I Did Yesterday, But I'm Not Sure About Tomorrow (Relationship Changes)

Sometimes I love my husband more than anything else in the world. I look at him with lust, thinking that not only is he the best partner for me, but also that I'm so lucky our paths crossed in that dodgy nightclub years ago. Other days, not only do I want to thump him if he breathes in the wrong way, but my anger bubbles up like uncontrollable vomit and makes gouging his eyes out seem like an acceptable option. If this happens to you, it's normal – just ensure anything you could use as a weapon is always more than an arm's length away.

So it's a given that cancer will change you, but it will also change everyone around you, the way you interact with them and how they interact with you. Some people will bolt as far away as possible, simply because they don't know how to handle it and are scared of getting close (perhaps your illness reminds them of a past bereavement not yet dealt with). Others will feel like they don't want to smother you. And others again will be your rock.

Isn't It All About Me!?

Well, it should be, but it's not going to go that way! Managing and navigating your way through your changing relationships can be tiring.

Helping Others Deal With Your Diagnosis

'Deborah will do what Deborah wants to do,' says my husband in annoyance during my overtly selfish periods. Now don't get me wrong – you are number one and the focus should be about getting through this. That will take up enough energy in itself. However, it was only after a while, when I really looked at some of the interesting behaviour of my children, that I realised that my cancer isn't just about me. More people than you realise will be affected by your cancer. Perhaps your parents are dealing with potentially losing a child, your siblings are worried about their mad big sister and your kids are living in fear that Mummy or Daddy might die. Have you stopped to think what sitting on the other side of the fence might feel like? How about the stark reality that says, for example, that my husband might be widowed before the age of 40 and left to play mum and dad alone? For some friends, your experience may be too close to home and may bring up a reminder of losing loved ones of their own, their own fears of immortality, their deep anxieties. I'm not expecting you to manage all these other people's emotions – but recognising that people will bring their own issues to the table, and might be deeply affected by them, can help both you and them sail through the process more smoothly.

Your friends and family will be amazing but don't be surprised if you notice a few of these characters popping up:

The over-emotional one	The one who can't handle it but still cares from afar	The one who is dealing with their own fears
'Oh this is all too sad!' They cry more than you and quite often you end up rubbing their back and telling them it will all be fine!	They sent you flowers when you were first diagnosed but seem to have disappeared in real life. However, they watch your Instagram stories every day and are the first to like any picture. They care – just in their own way.	You know it's tough for them as they only just sat through their mum's chemo last year.

The one who becomes obsessed with keeping you alive	The one who likes the attention too	The one who is there in every situation
Expect to be bombarded with the latest crazy cancer-related articles, not to mention deliveries of turmeric, hemp oil and every other weird and wonderful concoction!	Expect a few people to cling on to your story and act as your backstop. You will ultimately be grateful, and they will enjoy feeling like they are your special friend protecting you — make the most of it (if you can breathe!)	The solid rock who you know will just drop everything to be there. My mum and my sister are both this for me. Make sure you say thank you — often.
The one who makes things happen	**The one you get drunk with and who makes you laugh**	**The one you cry with**
You need the kids looking after, a lift to chemo, the dog walking. Before you've finished the conversation, it's happened. Yes please!	We love our wild child mate who will still be more interested in telling you about their latest relationship disasters as they smuggle Champagne on to the chemo ward than about worrying about what's going on with you. Cheers to that!	Get in the tissues, beers or ice cream, let your guard down and watch *Dirty Dancing*. They bring out the vulnerable side of you, listen with careful consideration and wipe your tears away afterwards.

You Need a Backstop

Find a friend or relative who has your back. Someone who will act as a personal assistant for all the admin tasks thrown at you, fight your corner and filter the updates back out to your circle of friends so you can choose only to deal with the ones you wish to. This may not be your partner but it does need to be someone close enough to know exactly what's going on and what help you might need at certain times.

Find Your Emotional Safe Place

Work out where you feel safe when you're in each mood. Who lifts you up the most? Where do you go for hope? Where for realism? Where to cry? You may be surprised – I was amazed by how often I ran 'home' to my parents.

Accept that not everyone will be positive. It's the nature of the beast and people around you will have had varied experiences of it.

Your Professional Friend

No one is ever too proud, important or strong to be above counselling help. Talking therapies and professional counselling, both group and individual, can provide you with a toolbox to cope with and navigate these changing relationships. Most hospitals will offer this as part of their services, but make sure you ask for it. Don't keep saying you are okay if you are struggling to find someone to talk to. Help is out there!

Being a Carer

So of course your world came crashing down when cancer entered, but if you are in a relationship so too did your partner's and your kids'. You need to be aware of that: the weight they also carry, the stress of knowing they are helpless in the situation, the extra household tasks they need to pick up, juggling the children between your good and bad days, the financial stress and the fear that one day they may be all alone, trying to put one foot in front of the other as they build Chapter 2 when they didn't want Chapter 1 to end.

I first met Stacey Heale through Instagram when her partner Greg was diagnosed with stage-four bowel cancer at the same time as me. With sheer determination she raised over £100K in just 48 hours to fund vital treatment.

My partner Greg was diagnosed with stage-four bowel cancer on our daughter's first birthday. Over the course of three days, he went from being told he had a particularly bad case of IBS to being informed that it was in fact inoperable cancer that had spread to his lungs. It's hard to explain the shock of news like that; terror, denial and rage all coursed through my body that night as I lay shaking between my parents in their bed. You do not expect to hear this news when you are 36 and have just started your family. I had a great career as a fashion academic and was due to return a week later after a year's maternity leave – my new work clothes were hanging up with tags still attached. I never got to wear them because, overnight, I became Greg's full-time carer and a stay-at-home mother to two children under the age of two.

There are a lot of new emotions that I have felt since Greg's diagnosis, and some of them are hard to recognise and admit. Sometimes I feel guilt that I am the healthy one. Sometimes I feel resentful that this is our life now and I've had to give up so much. Sometimes I feel the most overwhelming sadness that the dynamic of our relationship has changed, as is obvious when you take on the roles of patient and carer. I notice that I am angry more often and have less time for trivial problems. I am permanently exhausted, find it hard to focus, have a brain like a sieve and feel jealous of people planning holidays when I can't make plans more than two weeks in advance.

While in the past year all these feelings have surfaced, something else has grown in me too – a fierce determination to not let our lives be destroyed by cancer. I have so little control over what happens to Greg but I *do* have control over how I react to our situation. I realised quite early on that I could let cancer consume me or I could find a way to turn this shitstorm into something positive.

I became aware there were so few channels for people to discuss hard things going on in their lives. A long-time ignorer of social media, I did an about-turn and began writing my most vulnerable thoughts and feelings on Facebook. I used it as a vehicle to release my emotions out into the ether and I didn't expect the outpouring of connection and honesty I received back. Many of my posts went viral and my confession elicited responses; I began receiving private messages from countless strangers, confiding in me their most private thoughts. I didn't realise that becoming a carer would mean that my ability to care for all people would expand exponentially. Having a community where people could not feel alone seemed essential to me, as essential as the practical considerations of looking after Greg. A place like this proved impossible to find, so I created it myself. I started the website Beneath The

Weather as a place for essays on difficult topics, where others could contribute about the tough situations going on in their lives and create a dialogue. I had no idea what I was doing, nor had I even written anything before; but a reminder of mortality has a way of kicking you up the ass like nothing I've ever experienced.

Confessional narratives can seem self-indulgent and whiney but I feel it is critical to hear these voices, especially in the cancer world. There seem to be more voices of patients out there now, on places like Instagram, but I have struggled to find any carer role models to seek advice or solace from. If I were to give any advice, it would be to prioritise yourself. Yep, prioritise, as in you are number one. On paper, this might sound harsh and selfish but in reality, the opposite is true – no one can drink from an empty cup. If you are exhausted, rattled, stressed and on the edge, no amount of love you have for your family will make you able to look after them. You need time and space to rejuvenate so you can come back refreshed and ready to deal with whatever comes your way. Say yes to any help people want to offer you, whether that is food, taking the children out for an hour or coming to do your dishes. Pride will get you nowhere except fucking frazzled.

Just Pick Me Up Some Bread (How Can I Help You?)

Accept the fact that people will want to help you. Don't be backwards in coming forwards! People will say 'How can I help?' repeatedly. They will write it in cards, in texts, in emails – but 'help' might never come to fruition, simply because they don't know what to do and you don't either! Of course I am always flattered and humbled by the offers but it means I have to think of a way they could help me; and not only does it take brain cells to think of something, but when you've got serious chemo brain you can actually be very unsure of what you need. So I've outlined below a list, by category, of ways people can help you. You can wave this list in front of everybody as a starting point, but bear in mind that you may want to direct particular friend 'types' towards different things.

Logistics	— Drive me to chemotherapy/ radiotherapy/another appointment
	— Collect my prescriptions
	— Collect my children from school
	— Help me tidy my house
	— Can we spring-clean?

Keep me company	— Come to chemo with me
	— Come to a consultant appointment and write down what the doctor says
	— Visit me in hospital (I recommend this only for close friends and family)
	— Listen to me
	— Cry with me
Let's have fun	— Visit a nice garden or park for a walk
	— Go to the theatre
	— Go to the cinema
	— Cookery class
	— Meal out
	— Cocktail bar
	— Go shopping together
	— Sleepover night like we are 12 again!
Nurture me	— Deliver some meals
	— Cook for me
	— Send me a card
	— Sit and watch movies with me

Treat me (gift ideas)	— Arrange for a cleaner to come round
	— A flower subscription or nice plants for the garden
	— Buy me a nice candle
	— Take me to a spa for a day
	— Some nice slippers
	— Loungewear/PJs
	— A cosy blanket
	— Hot-water bottle
	— Get me a massage/reflexology voucher (but check treatment contraindications first)
	— A nice journal to write in
	— A photo album or frame
	— Chocolate, sweets and wine – always a winner!

Write to Me

This is so important – never underestimate the power of words.

The best presents I've ever received have been hand-written letters of motivation, love or just general nonsense to make me laugh. I have an ex-colleague who writes to me every few weeks. I didn't know her well when we worked together but what she does for me is amazing. She doesn't ask for anything in return but each time I receive a postcard I literally jump for joy. She tells me about her life, and what she's been up to, sends big love and good wishes and the whole thing makes me feel very special. Either hunt down a pen pal or drop very big hints to someone who enjoys writing about how much you love their letters.

Support and Relationships

TAKE-AWAY TOP TIPS

Here are the 'take-away' nuggets from this chapter to help you navigate those changing relationships:

Tip 1 Tell people in your own time – and decide how much you want them to know.

Tip 2 Have one key person who is the main communicator of your treatment updates.

Tip 3 You are not a burden – accept the help.

Tip 4 Get as much help as needed from charities and hospital services.

Tip 5 Take a moment to think how your carer and those closest to you are coping – get them help if needed.

Tip 6 Accept that your relationships with most people will change – in bad ways and good ways.

Tip 7 Write letters – it's good for the mind and soul.

• • •

'Love those who will love you when you have
nothing to offer but your company.'

Anonymous

Chapter 6

Uncle C is Coming to Stay – Be Polite, I Know He Smells!

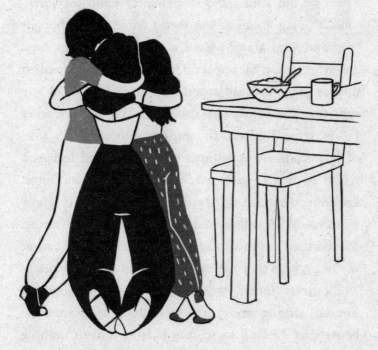

Telling Your Children (The Hardest Thing I've Ever Done)

Do you have children? Straight after diagnosis, did your mind immediately jump to worrying about telling them? Mine did. I thought long and hard about what I wanted to tell them, how and when and what impact it might have. How on earth do you get your head around telling children – of any age – that Mum or Dad has cancer? Having been a teacher for 15 years, I've seen the impact from 'the other side' of how children of all ages can behave and feel as a result of things such as cancer going on at home. Choosing what and when you tell your children is totally up to you. A lot will depend on the age of your offspring. Maybe they are too young to even know what cancer is – or perhaps they have grown up and flown the nest.

I'll never forget, when my doctors first found a tumour, drying my eyes and walking back into the house that evening to see the kids as though nothing had happened. I didn't want to drag them into my blind panic and worry until I knew what was happening to me. I'd recommend waiting to tell your children until you know exactly what you have and what the treatment plan involves. They will ask you questions and being able to respond with clear-cut answers will reduce the worry for them. I therefore chose to tell my children (eight and ten at the time of writing) from the day we knew for sure it was cancer and let them get involved in what was going on with my treatment. This felt right for us, and for their ages – and seeing as I'd be going through lots of different procedures and changing my whole daily routine and work, it would have been impossible to hide it. Soon enough they would have been asking questions and trying to fill in the gaps themselves – which I'm sure would have meant they'd be jumping to the worst conclusions and speculating over what might be. Research does however show that children under the age of five, while they may pick up on a change of emotions, won't really understand what cancer is – and I know many mums in this position who have just said 'Mummy is poorly' and haven't used the big C word.

Children's reactions to cancer and what they understand will depend on their age and this may determine what you choose to share with your little or not-so-little ones:

- **Babies and toddlers** won't understand what's happening. Keeping their routines familiar when possible will help.

- **Children aged three to five** won't fully understand the cancer. But they will notice changes to emotions and routines. They might think wishing can make things happen, or that your illness is their fault. They may also become clingy. Keeping to routines, reassuring them that the cancer isn't their fault and setting boundaries can help.

- **Children aged six to 12** will understand more about cancer. They might not tell you their fears. You may notice changes in their behaviour. Let them help out and make sure they keep up with school and friends.

- **Teenagers** usually understand the cancer but may not want to talk. They might want to help out more, but also want their independence. Encouraging them to ask questions, asking their opinion and giving them space when they want it can help.

(Source: Macmillan)

When Do I Tell Them?

I worked myself up for days over how my children might react when I told them. Would they just break down and cry? And how would I cope with that? But the thought of it was actually worse than the reality.

In reality I got two inquisitive children, who were obviously concerned but who, after all their questions were answered, said 'So Mummy, because you'll be around more, can you pick me up from school tomorrow in the car?'

What are the key things to include when telling children? Some of the pointers in the table below should help:

Use the correct words and explain them if needed – bowel cancer, chemotherapy, radiotherapy. You may need to repeat things often for younger children.	Be honest and don't make promises. My kids said 'Are you going to be okay?' – I said 'The doctors are going to do everything they possibly can to ensure I am.'	Let them ask questions and lots of them. Spend 15 minutes with paper and pen writing them all down and answer them one by one.

| Explain to them if there will be practical changes in the way life looks – for example, I suddenly went from working full-time to being around more. Perhaps other people will collect them from school. But reassure them that their routine will stay the same as much as possible. | Ask children for help. Don't put pressure on them, but giving them little jobs to do around the house will help them feel useful. My children really enjoy making me breakfast in bed at the weekends (– it's a win–win as long as they don't make too much of a mess in the process!). | Try to tell them about some positives. For example – 'Because Mummy will be tired we get to have more movie nights together! Yay!'. Or 'You'll get to see lots more of Grandma and Grandad.' |

Where Do I Say It?

It is important to choose a place to tell your children where you know they are comfortable. Following advice from a good friend, we went to a local restaurant that we often go to, for a few reasons:

- Seeing Mummy crying might upset children. In public in a restaurant, you may be less likely to do it. There is nothing wrong with crying, of course, but they might get more upset if they see you upset.
- It stops them running off into their bedrooms and hiding under the covers.

- It means that the initial, horribly difficult, conversation can end when you leave the restaurant, and life can continue as 'normal' when you get back home.
- A glass of wine and good food puts the adults in a better mood!

Prepare Them as Much as Possible

When we are not prepared for something and are off guard, we might find things harder to deal with. Children will judge how you are doing based on the way you act and look, so if this is going to change tell them! My daughter found it very hard visiting me in hospital after an operation as we hadn't prepared her for the fact that Mummy was going to have tubes and leads coming out. She became fascinated by the catheter pot of wee and the stomach drain, to the point that it's her only memory of Mummy in hospital. She was quite freaked out by it and as a result is now a little apprehensive about hospital visits. The following operation, we ensured that all my leads and tubes were out before she visited and this certainly helped.

Ensure that you tell your children what will happen as far as possible – for example, if you are going to have an operation and it will leave scars, perhaps show them what the scars might look like; or, if you will lose your hair, why not show them pictures of other people who have and get them to choose a nice headscarf with you if that's going to be your thing. I carry a portable chemo pump around for two days of each cycle and it was important that the children understood how the chemo pump plays an important role in giving me my medicine. I also warned them they needed to be bit more careful around Mummy so as not to knock it! Once I understood how the pumps worked myself, I showed them pictures online of what mine might look like and we talked about it. This gave them an opportunity to ask questions.

Hugo and Eloise's Advice Corner! Only Kids Allowed!

I asked my little monsters Eloise, eight, and Hugo, ten, to share some advice straight from the horse's mouth that you can use to help your own kids.

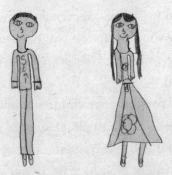

Drawn by Eloise (aged eight)

Questions we asked mummy:

- Will you be ok?

- Is your cancer dangerous?

- What's the name of your cancer?

- Will I see you more often?

- What will happen to you?

- What is chemotherapy?

- What happens if the medicine doesn't work?

- How many operations do you think you will have?

- Will you lose your hair?

- Will you be very sick?

'It's ok to feel sad and scared sometimes. But stay strong — you can get through this'
Eloise

• • •

Below is a list of things that my kids suggest could be used to help you. Why not show this to your children and let them pick a few to try each week?

Things you can do to help (Written by Hugo and Eloise)

- Fetch Mummy or Daddy stuff when they ask for it – Mummy normally asks for tissues and chocolate.
- Give them lots of hugs – they need it.
- Read a book together.
- Sometimes your Mummy or Daddy will be really tired so just curl up together and watch a good movie – we LOVE movie night!
- Try to get your school stuff ready on time so they don't need to shout – we are bad at this!
- Ask Mummy to buy you weird things online sometimes after she has chemo – we get funny things because the drugs Mummy has make her a bit silly! My favourite was the cheese toastie-maker!
- Have fun together! We dance after each chemo session to celebrate. One of us designs the dance moves and one of us sorts the clothes! We even film them and put them on Instagram!

Hugo and Eloise's Words of Wisdom!

- Ask lots of questions.
- Don't be afraid. Cancer is scary but not always.
- Always have hope — doctors can do some really good things.
- If you need to have a cry that's okay.
- Tell people how you are feeling, especially if you are finding it very hard.

When my Mummy got Cancer by Hugo Poland Bowen (aged ten)

It was scary when I found out that Mummy had cancer. I felt frightened and lots of other feelings, like being scared of being alone. I had lots of questions because I had never encountered cancer before. My first thoughts were — are you going to be okay? And what will happen to you? Knowing Mummy had cancer made me worry. I felt anxious and nervous about what might happen. I also felt a bit angry that my Mummy had cancer and other mummies didn't. Why my Mummy?

I asked lots of questions about the cancer and they made me feel sad because it's just a sad feeling to know that your Mum has cancer.

Lots of things changed when Mummy got cancer — like I saw more of her and she started a blog. Mummy was really tired and couldn't do as many activities and I felt unhappy. It was scary when Mummy had operations because you didn't know what would happen. I was nervous about what chemotherapy would do — I thought she would be on edge and crazy. There are some positives. I have enjoyed seeing Mummy more and I enjoy some of the activities she gets us into. Also I enjoy doing our chemo dances and I like doing events to raise money for cancer charities. I'm proud when I see Mummy on TV or listen to her on the radio. For the future I hope that Mummy's cancer goes away and it doesn't come back but that Mummy is still around more. I also hope that the world can find lots of new cures so that nobody needs to be worried about cancer any more.

When my Mummy got Cancer by Eloise Poland Bowen (aged eight)

When I found out I was nervous. My question was 'Are you going to lose your hair?' I was scared that she was going to die. The thing that changed in my life was that I am always scared.

The bad things were that Mummy was always tired when she was on chemo. I did not like seeing Mummy when she had the pee bag in hospital because it was gross — just imagine having a massive bag on the side of your bed that is full of pee and a tube that you wee into. In hospital I like riding on the chairs.

The good things about Mummy getting cancer are that she is around more and that she is not always working. All my friends ask me how I am so I'm quite popular. I am very proud of Mummy for keeping strong and not giving up. Sometimes Mummy does crying moments and sometimes not. I enjoy doing photographs with Mummy and dancing. For the future I want Mummy to live and to be able to wear her shoes.

Supporting Your Children

What are some of the practical things you can do to help your children through this difficult period?

Give Them Something to Look Forward To

Depending on your course of treatment, it's often nice to give children something to look forward to, perhaps when treatment is over or if a break from chemotherapy is on the horizon. For example, a holiday when treatment is over, a camping trip or a party while you're on a break – why not let them decide! I wouldn't set it in stone – and don't make promises you don't think you can keep – but I'd certainly talk to them about things you will do together and when. If you are in a position where your treatment plan is just one step at a time, let them celebrate each milestone with you – perhaps with a day trip out, a visit to a museum or a walk in your favourite park. Remember milestones can be anything from another chemo cycle done, a stable scan or getting through an operation to just getting to a Friday and celebrating that it's the weekend.

Keep a Sense of Normality

As far as possible, keep things normal for them. Stick to the same routine, keep the same childcare (if it still works for you) and act as though life will just continue in the same way – to a point.

Visiting You in Hospital

Only allow your children to visit you once you have prepared them in terms of what they might see. As I mentioned earlier, my daughter got quite scared when first visiting me. If I know that I'm having a small procedure with maybe only a night's stay, I now don't tell my children until after it has happened so as not to worry them. There is no need for them to visit me so I don't wish to put them through the extra stress.

Pen Pals

Encourage your children to write, if they are old enough. This may be in a diary, to a relative, a godparent, a friend or to yourself. This can provide a fantastic way for them to express how they are feeling. The more old-school you go with this the better, in my opinion – writing an email doesn't have the same effect, or allow you to sit and explore how you are really feeling, as does having to take time to handwrite a letter. You'll be pleasantly surprised sometimes what they write. I was really worried about my daughter and how she was coping – she, however, was more worried about what outfit she would wear to the school disco! I've never laughed so much as when we were on a woodland Christmas walk and arrived at the 'wishing tree' station. My son melted my heart by attaching a label to the tree that wished for Mummy to not have cancer... and my daughter attached one that wished for a pony!

It's Good to Talk!

The more you can talk about your cancer and normalise it as part of your life, the less scared your children will be. It will enable them to feel safe about asking questions if they feel they need to. You may not be the person they wish to talk to – they may prefer a grandparent, a friend, a relative. If you know that your child prefers talking with someone else, arm that person with the facts so they can relay an accurate picture of your health and your treatment.

We Are Family

You may find that cancer brings you closer together as a family. You may take great comfort from knowing that your kids are right behind you as your number one cheerleaders. On those bad days, when you start questioning why you are putting your body through chemotherapy, you may just find that an evening spent curled up together provides you with the strength required to get through the next cycle.

Get Help

Lots of organisations can provide help for you and your children, including your GP, social workers and local counselling services – and also please refer to the resources at the back. It's really important to let the school know what is going on as quite often children may be fine at home but act out of character at school. As a teacher, I know it was quite common for children to really act up if things were going on at home. Be warned that 'acting up' might not look like a raging argument with smashing pots. Instead watch for changes in behaviour – this could be anything from trying to push boundaries to not complying with behaviour rules or suddenly changing friendship groups (a way of looking for attention).

Schools quite often offer counselling services, and pupils may choose to talk to teachers about what's going on at home. It's important that the school is informed with the correct information so they can support your child in the right way.

Making Memories Today To Last a Lifetime

Cancer can all too often become the main focus at home – but not only does life need to go on, children need to see a life beyond cancer. They are likely to have to endure a change in logistics and see you looking poorly, as well as facing and dealing with their own fears. But just because you are worried about your future doesn't mean their daily life needs to plummet into sadness and panic. Having special, fun and memorable things to focus on with your kids can distract them (and you) from thinking about the big C word and focusing on making memories can play a huge part in flipping the experience, as far as possible, into a positive one.

Making memories is not about packing your life into a box in the hope that it will never need to be opened. It's about making the most of each and every moment – as we should do anyway. It should allow you an opportunity to reassess what you and your family value most and how you wish to live moving forwards, to think about celebrating the small milestones and looking towards the future with hope. Perhaps for many people it is a little wake-up call about what's truly important.

The first advice given to me when I found out that my cancer had metastasised was to make a memory box for each child. A memory box is a collection of items, letters and other objects or photographs that represent you. While the concept of this kind of memory box has its uses (and yes, I do encourage you to look into them), to me the idea felt very mechanical – an exercise in trying to represent me in a shoebox – and to be honest the idea just made me feel sad. Also, I felt I wanted my children to remember me (when I'm very old and my time is up) and their childhood through the way I made them feel, the personality traits they have, the traditions we created and the experiences we shared, as opposed to items I've placed in a box.

Your diagnosis may just act as a catalyst to ensure you book the family holiday you've always wanted to, take on the challenge of a lifetime or ensure things are in order for your children long-term. You might as a family choose to take a look at how you really want to live and what makes things special for you – regardless of what the future may hold. For me, my wake-up call has set me off on a mission to make memories today that will last a lifetime. And while we'd all love an unlimited purse and a round-the-world trip, for me it's the little things and traditions that I want my children to continue to love – cancer or no cancer.

Start with Your Best Memories and the Rest will Follow

People always make bucket lists of things they just have to do – but why not celebrate all the things you've already done?! Sit down with your children, partner or friends and mind-map what are your favourite memories to date and why. As a starting point, why not use the following questions:

What's the best experience we've ever had?
What's the best trip or holiday we've ever been on?
What's your favourite thing to do at home?
When are you the happiest?
What days and things do you look most forward to?
Who do you most like spending time with?
What do you enjoy doing most at weekends?
What's your funniest memory (perhaps of the person with cancer) to date?
If you had a free day and unlimited money what would you do?

For each question, discuss why you enjoy it and how it makes you feel. And decide as a family if you'd like to do this more often or not. I did this with my children and I was pleasantly surprised to find out that it's not always the big expensive holidays that give them their favourite memories – it can be a favourite book you read to them, or games you play around the dinner table, or that time when the dog ran away and you spent hours hunting him down.

Don't Write a Bucket List, Write a Life List!

A bucket list, by nature, conjures up a 'to-do list' that must be done just to say 'I've been there and got the T-shirt.' Now I don't know about you, but my to-do list normally stays as a list and never really comes to fruition. Things stay on it for months and nothing ever happens!

So instead think of your list as a life list and use it as an opportunity to look at the changes you wish to make, the things you wish to try out and the things you want to stop doing in your life. And make sure it happens – NOW.

Things I wish to continue and do more of	Things I wish to try out	Things I want to give up and stop in my life	In the future our life will look like ...

So let me outline my top five key suggestions and ideas you could try to create a home full of memories rather than a home full of cancer:

1. *Alphabet cancer celebrations*

There will be good days, and using these means that you can save your energy and put it into making some memories! The concept of alphabet activities came to me when a friend suggested I tried alphabet dating – and no, it's not about dating men for each letter, although that could be another creative use of the game! The idea is that you list activities for each letter and pick a letter at random each time you want to do something or celebrate. I tried an alphabet summer holiday with my children a few years back and they loved it. They had so much fun coming up with the activities for the grid. I've given you some suggestions as a starting point – but what will your alphabet grid include?

A: Art gallery	B: Bowling	C: Camping	D: Dancing	E: Exploring	F: Frisbee
G: Golf	H: Hiking	I: Ice cream	J: Jazz night	K: Kite-flying	L: Lunch out
M: Museum	N: Night out	O: Opera	P: Picnic	Q: Quiz	R: Road trip
S: Seaside	T: Theatre	U: Up! (Why not take a hot-air balloon ride!)	V: Visit friends	W: Walk	X: X marks the spot! (treasure hunt)
Y: Yes day	Z: Zoo				

2. *Creating traditions*

Traditions don't need to cost money, and they don't need to be overthought. They could be as simple as a game you always play at dinner, the way you read a story at night-time or the way Santa leaves sacks in a particular place. Traditions are easy-to-pick-up ideas that children will recall and which they might even follow with their children in the future. Some we have in our family include:

- Treasure hunts, especially around Easter time. These have got more and more complex as the kids have grown up and now they even create their own for each other and for me.
- Movie nights with popcorn – it's a good way to make watching a movie feel special.
- Mealtime games – my husband is obsessed with playing games such as 'Just a Minute' and the 'Yes/No game'.
- A lazy tooth fairy who never arrives on time and leaves hilarious notes!
- Key events each year that you look forward to – every year I go overboard on Halloween.
- Mummy likes to throw a party – it's true, I do. Each year we have a summer party and a winter party. The children really enjoy this as they get to run riot for no apparent reason.

I suspect you'll find you already have things that are traditions in your family. Even when you are undergoing treatment, do try to keep these things up – not only will it make you feel better, it will make your kids feel like everything is running normally.

3. *Say cheese!*
My family are officially fed up that I take pictures at every opportunity. For me, however, photos both good and bad capture my children growing up and remind me of all the fabulous times we spend together. I choose not to print my photos but to document them through my Instagram account, almost using it as an album in itself. While you need to ensure that photo-taking doesn't take over the moment, you will never look back and regret the photos you took of your life. Set up an online memory photo bank (this could just be a Google Drive). Photo books now are accessible and easy to make from websites such as www.photobox.co.uk – commit to make one, once a month for a year throughout your treatment – and why not continue it into recovery! It will enable your children to see the positive things you did during that time.

4. *Have a ticket box or a cork bucket*
Why not try having one of these in your house?

Ticket Box	Cork Bucket
Have a box that all the family know about. Each time you visit a theme park, or your favourite museum, for example, keep one of the entry tickets to put in the box. It's lovely every so often to go through the tickets and recall the fun times you all had at each venue.	Each time you crack open a bottle of fizzy or other nice wine, keep the cork and write the occasion on it. I have friends who now have massive jars filled with corks from each occasion they've celebrated over the years – you will, however, realise just how much wine you've drunk!

5. *Emails to the future*
Set up email accounts for your children from a young age and write to them. I did this when they were born and gave the address to family members and close friends. In the children's early years I asked people to send them email messages and pictures of things that they liked or activities they did together. It meant that when my children took over their email accounts recently, they had a bank of messages from loved ones telling them about their early years. You can use it to send emails to your future self and for other people as well as your children:

- Email your future self, reminding you how brave you are being.
- Email your children letters for their futures – 'To be opened on your sixteenth birthday'/'Your wedding day'/'Your first day at university'.
- Why not set up an account for your friend or relative with cancer? Ask people to email motivational quotes, funny stories or memories to a new email account that the person undergoing treatment can read when they are feeling low.

Fertility and Cancer

I was taken aback in my first oncologist meeting when he asked if I wanted more children. My husband and I immediately turned to each other and said 'No.' My oncologist said, 'Do you need time to think about this?' and we both responded again with a firm 'No.' I could see the relief on my husband's face that the conversations we'd been having previously regarding a third child were now totally off the agenda. I got excited that dog conversations were back on... And sure enough a cute little cavapoo named Winston duly followed!

For the majority of cancer patients, losing fertility as a result of treatment isn't an issue, whether that's because they are already going through menopause or because they simply don't want to have any more children. Personally, I wanted to get on with treatment and be around for my current children more than I wanted the option of having more. Some people, however, and maybe you are one of them, may not have had children yet or may be wanting to have more. While not all chemotherapy or treatment plans will render you infertile, do ensure you ask. And ensure you are offered options to freeze your eggs or sperm should you wish to do so. Most hospitals will organise this quickly so as not to interfere or delay your treatment too much, but you will have to go through a series of procedures to ensure the best chance of good-quality embryos/sperm/eggs being stored. Make sure you take time to decide what to do. I've met many people who chose not to give themselves the option of preserving their fertility and have regretted it at a later date. If you have any concerns or questions over fertility issues please speak to your healthcare team, who can advise you on options available.

Uncle C is Coming to Stay

TAKE-AWAY TOP TIPS

Here are the 'take-away' nuggets from this chapter to help you navigate and support your children through your diagnosis:

Tip 1   Remember that the way children react will vary according to their age.

Tip 2   Being open and honest will stop them filling in the gaps and jumping to the worst conclusion.

Tip 3   Prepare them for your treatment by talking them through what might happen to you and what they might notice.

Tip 4   Flip the home attitude and environment from dealing with cancer to making memories: have moments today that will make memories tomorrow to last a lifetime.

Tip 5   Cancer treatment might affect your fertility – ensure you ask this question before you start treatment and find out what options are available to you.

Chapter 7

Where Will I Find Shoes to Match My Chemo Pump? Looking Good and Feeling Better

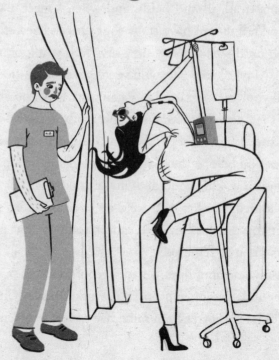

The Power of Looking Good

I have found that throughout my treatment, I've become more interested in the way I look and how it affects my daily mood. I want to look 'normal'. I don't want to look like the images portrayed of cancer patients (frail, ill and bald), and when I meet a stranger and tell them I have stage-four cancer, I secretly pat myself on the back when they say 'Well you look really well.' Maybe, like me, you've always made 'looking good' your business, and you can't see why you should stop that now just because cancer has arrived – why drop the lippy, the heels, the sharp suits? If they were a part of you before, they can and should still be a part of you now. Looking good does make you feel better – if it were a medicine I'm sure we'd be overdosing on it! So add it to your kicking-arse cancer toolbox and pull it out as often as required!

In my teaching days, I had a reputation for pushing the boundaries of appropriate 'work dress'. 'Girls, if your skirt is shorter than mine, we have a problem,' I'd declare, running around the school in five-inch stilettos and a slightly-too-tight bright green dress. An amazing head teacher who I trained under would declare that 'Any occasion is only as good as the way you dress for it. Look scruffy, and your mind will become scruffy.' While I know I was naughty walking the fine line between making school an important business occasion and treating it like a fun evening out, getting dressed in the morning was certainly an event in itself! Putting on make-up, and making an effort to become 'presentable' to the world, worked wonders in lifting my mood each day. It ensured my head was in the game and perhaps put a smile on others' faces when I'd argue that my hot-pink dress was indeed acceptable 'business attire'!

Looking smart was something I took for granted – it was just part of me and what I did each day. That was until along with my diagnosis came a break in my teaching career. For various reasons, I couldn't continue being a teacher on the front line, and with that break came a break from the daily routine of getting dressed up and donning the highest heels I could run in. At first I welcomed an excuse to slob around in pyjamas (that I'd try to pull off as regular trousers), and to walk down the high street in them matched with my husband's over-sized jumpers. But then came the lack of caring whether my hair was washed... and before I knew it, I was well and truly a 20-year-old university student in the body of a 35-year-old who couldn't even be bothered to get out of bed!

Now, before I get shouted down, looking good doesn't mean having to look like you've just stepped off the catwalk. Good is whatever makes YOU feel nice. We are all allowed days where we don't get dressed – the kind when you watch back-to-back episodes of *Friends* and order takeaway. And let's face it, when you are undergoing treatment you don't need any excuses to have those days. But over the course of my treatment I noticed a clear correlation between the days when I'd made an effort to 'look better' and the buoyancy of my mood. For me 'looking good' is more of a feeling inside – and despite loving a bright red lippy, I can sometimes feel my best with no make-up on, in wellies and yoga pants! Perhaps for you it's in your walking gear, perhaps it's in some nice PJs – but the thing I want you to ask is when do you feel most 'alive' and ready to take on the day?

On what I'd consider 'better days', I popped on some make-up, and made a little effort – not five-inch-heel type effort but maintenance basics – clean underwear and clothes that I could leave the house in! As a result, it was on those days that I did leave the house, and I certainly felt more upbeat. In contrast, the days when I couldn't lift my head off the pillow, let alone change my underwear (yes, you too will have these days!), were my roughest. We all must of course listen to our bodies and take it easy when we need to, but I often found that even when I started the day thinking that all I would have the energy to do was close my eyes, roll over and go back to sleep, it was in fact a shower, some clean clothes and a good splattering of lippy and a walk that made me feel better.

Fake It Until You Feel It!

Let me tell you a little story that I believe is a good metaphor for how you might approach the question of 'are you ready to face the day and all it throws at you?' I'll refer you back to the wise words of my previous boss – 'any occasion is only as good as the way you dress for it'. Why not make having the gift of life an occasion in itself? Get out your Sunday best, bring out the sequins or slap on the bright red lipstick; whatever makes you feel good. Men, shine those shoes and dust down your sharpest jacket – dressing well might just be the ammunition you need to get you through the rough days. If you are like me, when I look in the mirror, if I look rough, I feel rough. However, peer in the mirror and look 'okay', even if I'm hidden behind a barrage of smart clothes and make-up, I can almost kid myself into believing that I've got this. You too may find that kidding yourself may just be enough to make it become a reality. Trust me – go stand in front of the mirror, no lippy or heels (or whatever are your weapons of choice) and shout 'Fuck you cancer!' Then do it with a face full of make-up and your favourite stilettos and tell me you don't feel more empowered!

But I'm Not a Dressing-up Kind of Person

Does wellies on a Wednesday and jeans every day fit more with your take on 'dressing for the occasion'? Great! I'm not suggesting we all start dressing as though we want to audition for *Ru Paul's Drag Race* – what I'm getting at is putting your self-care at the forefront of your mind and ensuring that you're taking time to feel good about yourself. Ask yourself – what makes me feel good and confident? Is it newly washed hair, a favourite shirt or clean nails? Beauty and confidence is all about what's inside... but I have to add, if you are anything like me, you might sometimes need the mascara to help bring it out.

My Shopping Habit

It's a running joke in my house that I'm having an affair with my postman. We do chat most days, him awkwardly (because I'm usually half-dressed) delivering yet another one of the weird and wonderful finds that I accidently bought while away with the fairies during my latest chemotherapy treatment! Be prepared – it's all too easy when lying on the sofa feeling delirious to start adding things into your virtual basket, and before you know it, it will have arrived at your front door!

This is a warning (mainly to myself, admittedly) – watch that shopping habit. The last thing you'll need after you have kicked the cancer is to find yourself with a bunch of 'things' you no longer want because they just remind you of treatment, not to mention a big credit card bill to pay off. Why not try to stick (mostly) to window-shopping instead? But you can have some fun regardless of budget – and you know what, if anyone deserves it, you do!

Any Excuse!

'I've got cancer' is the only excuse you need to justify buying that glittery dress you've been eyeing up for a while – even if it's just to wear to your next chemo. I strongly believe that trekking around the shops and doing lots of outfit changes actually counts as exercise – or at least that's what I've been telling myself for years. But there are some genuine reasons that you might need to take a little trip to the shops; or, if you are like my husband and completely allergic to shopping, then having a splurge online while sipping a glass of red might be more up your street.

From workwear to loungewear	You may find that your wardrobe needs a temporary makeover. Is it full of suits and heels? As fun as it can be to wear your favourite high heels during a chemo session, you will probably crash afterwards. You can feel just as glam in some good loungewear or PJs; depending on budget, invest in the best-quality, nicest items you can. It's essential that you have spare sets; you may be surprised at just how many clean sets are required in a day if you're having a rough period. And yes, there will be times when you feel like a nappy and towel would be the best solution.
New scars	Are you the proud owner of some new body art?! Perhaps you have some keyhole scars, or perhaps like me you are collecting what looks like bites across your body. Either way, scars need to be taken care of and existing clothes can rub them. For example, I needed higher and looser waistbands for a while to cope with my large stomach scar, and after my lung operation my bras rubbed. Now that's an excuse for new clothes if ever there was one!

Colostomy bags	Do you have a new bag? One of those you can't find in the fancy-pants Bond Street stores?! Like me and many of my fellow 'Bowelies', dressing to accommodate your new 'poo bag' may mean for you a shift in waistlines, darker clothing in the early days until you get used to your new friend and underwear that helps you feel supported. Don't worry — with a few adjustments you can rock a colostomy bag and still look smoking!
New boobs	You may have gone shopping for new boobs already, or maybe you are getting used to your one-boob wonder? Either way, if you have undergone breast surgery you will need to get a well-fitting bra. Find specialist help and get measured properly. Debenhams and Marks & Spencer both offer this service — just go to your local branch and ask.
Because I just want to feel nice!	Sometimes you just need to feel nice about yourself. Embrace the idea of hunting for a new outfit for a special occasion, perhaps a friend's birthday party, a wedding or a cancer celebratory night out. You deserve it!

Brighten Your Life and Accessorise!

I'm a little black dress kind of girl. Or, in loungewear terms, black leggings and a black T-shirt. But often I find that adding a bit of colour brightens up a dark day – especially while I'm sitting in that chemo chair. If you don't feel comfortable dressing head to toe in bright orange, then accessories are your new best friend. You can transform a plain black dress with a striking bright red necklace, or add statement earrings to the most boring of outfits – you'll be ready to take on the world. Fuck you, chemo!

> **Tip!** Ladies listen up! I cannot urge you enough to book yourself into one of the free workshops run by the lovely people at Look Good Feel Better. Two hours of dedicated 'you' time, fab conversation with other patients in a secure environment and a goody bag of make-up dreams – I guarantee you will look good and feel better! Look Good Feel Better (LGFB) is the only international cancer support charity that helps women and teenagers manage the visible side effects of cancer treatment. Their aim is to greatly increase people's confidence and self-esteem at a very difficult time in their lives. For more information visit **www.lookgoodfeelbetter.co.uk**

Face the day

You know what you are going to be met with when you look in the mirror, right? With me, it's normally a tired and older version of someone who used to look 20... But what happens when you are scared to look in the mirror because you know you won't recognise the reflection in front of you? Perhaps it's hair loss, maybe it's the moon face from steroids or scars from operations, but suddenly it's not the 'you' you know. While we can't stop these physical changes, we can, armed with the right ammunition, learn to be confident with them.

Styling Out the Changes

Regardless of the intricacies of each drug and its side effects, there are common things that are likely to change for most people undergoing treatment. So how do you style them out?

Skin:	Nails:
Depending on your drugs, your skin may break out with teenage acne or look like a flaky snowfall of dryness. It may become sore and red.	Most chemotherapy regimes will make your nails dry, brittle and weak. Fingertips may become sore and skin around the nail edge is more likely to become inflamed.
Tip: Invest in some good-quality skincare products and get into a skincare routine. Many brands or counters in department stores will offer free skin consultations and testers and some even specialise in people going through cancer treatment. I used a Dermalogica range specifically designed for very sensitive skin.	**Tip:** Ladies, even if you were not previously a nail varnish wearer – become one. Prepare to go vampish! The rumour mill on the chemo ward is that dark nail varnish will offer protection from these side effects, and you know what – in my experience it sure does work.

Tiredness:	Body aches:
Feeling tired during treatment is a given, and you will need plenty of rest, but it can be styled out so you don't feel like a complete slob.	Is your body in a constant state of aches and pains? For many the combination of a reduction in activity and drug side effects can make you feel as though you've hiked up a mountain, when really you just rolled over in bed. Stiffness and soreness might be your new norm.
Tip: Invest in some good 'chilling at home clothes', or 'loungewear' as they're otherwise known. The kind of stuff that you still feel comfortable in but can change into from your PJs and feel stylish. Go retro and snap up a few matching loungewear twinsets. When you walk the dog, no one will know you've just had a snooze in the same clothes!	**Tip:** Get a massage. Many hospitals now offer them as part of their complementary therapy services. You could ask your partner or a friend to perform one, but it's advisable to get it done by someone who specialises in massage for people in treatment. It's a sure-fire way to make you feel better and relax and reinvigorate those muscles all at the same time.

Indulge Your Inner Goddess

'But I don't have time!' Well, ladies and gentlemen, now is the moment in your life to make time. You know that list of priorities you have? Looking after yourself needs to get higher up there. If you are not functioning then nothing else will happen anyway, so start being a little bit selfish. Your body may not be a temple, but my word it's taking a battering and needs rewarding, relaxation and a bit of well-deserved TLC. This includes getting your nails done, having a facial (although be careful to find a specialist who understands the sensitivity of your skin) and lighting some candles, getting into a hot bath, pouring yourself a glass of good wine and locking the bathroom door.

How to Style a Chemo Pump

'You wear high heels to chemo?' asked my astonished friend. Well yes, actually sometimes I do! And other times I dress in an orange jumpsuit – and other times in whichever kick-arse slogan T-shirt I've come across most recently. But you can go either way here. I was given this tip, which works really well for lots of people to help put their chemo behind them and move on:

> Why not buy a comfy outfit, one you don't care too much for and that's not very expensive, and wear it to every chemo session? At the end of chemo take great pleasure in throwing it away!

As well as how you choose to dress for chemo, you can take a barrage of things with you to make you feel more comfortable – here are my top five:

- Big cosy socks to change into for the session.
- A bobble hat – normally chemo makes you feel cold, so this will make you feel snuggly.
- A small blanket. Hospitals do provide you with blankets, but there is nothing like your own one.
- Some bright lipstick or your favourite lip balm. Looking good may be the last thing on your mind, but I promise you, if you're anything like me a slick of lipstick after you have vomited will make you feel less depressed when you stare at your grey reflection in the mirror! Think of the nice smell of a new lipstick with that glistening look shouting 'just wear me – I will cheer you up no end' – and a bit of moisture on your dry lips will help to ease the side effects of sitting for too long in an air-conditioned hospital!
- Face moisturiser – the air conditioning will make your skin feel dry. And your hands will be grateful for a little massage while you are rubbing it in.

Coping With Hair Loss

Do any of these questions and concerns sound familiar?

- I don't want to look like I have cancer.
- My head is a funny shape and a wig just won't suit me.

- I may never end treatment or get a break and I don't want to die bald.
- I don't want to see myself in the mirror with no hair – I won't be me.
- What happens if I wear a wig and it falls off in public?
- I don't want to scare my children.
- It makes my cancer too visibly real and I'm not ready for that.

Let me take a punt here – did you used to assume that everyone who's on chemotherapy ends up bald?

I honestly thought that cancer always equalled hair loss. I soon learned, when I started my first regime of chemotherapy, that this was well and truly a myth. In fact, looking around the room on my first treatment, I saw that more people had hair than didn't! But the idea scared me to the point that I still don't know how I would cope if I had to have drugs that guaranteed I'd go bald. To show you just how much this frightened me – I didn't have the typical reaction when I was told that my cancer had spread to my lungs. Rather than my first question being 'am I going to die?' it was 'am I going to lose my hair?' When I was told there was a good chance I would, it took a lot of convincing on the healthcare team's side and research on mine to persuade me to go ahead with the new regime.

I was not alone – and, if you're frightened of this, neither are you; research suggests that 8 per cent of cancer patients refuse chemotherapy because of the fear of losing their hair.

But It's Only Hair…

A good hair day makes me feel feminine and sexy – flick it in the right way and I'm ready to go into battle! Perhaps I'm making up for my teenage years of under-cuts and pixie crops, but I'm now rather in love with my hair – wavy with a good amount of schoolgirl frizz – even though I spent most of my younger years cursing it in the hunt for straighteners to tame the beast! So telling me 'it's just hair' is like telling me to not care about my left arm – or right leg for that matter!

Okay, so there are some brave souls, and maybe you are one of them, who throw caution to the wind, get out the razor and cry 'well, it will grow back anyway!' They rock the look with pride and look damn good on it.

I was never going to be one of those people. It may be 'only hair', but for some of us it's a security net, another barrier we can use to look like we don't have cancer. It may be the last remaining shield we feel protected by, and we might fear that if that breaks then we break. Having these feelings is totally normal and yes, it's okay to plan for not wanting to look at a bald you. It's okay to be 'vain' and admit to feeling unhappy about your impending loss.

Audrey is a friend of mine through social media – she documented her breast cancer journey through her blog *Cancer With a Smile*.

Hair loss is one of the first things people associate with cancer. That big shiny napper is like a beacon shouting 'Look at me, I've got cancer!' to the world. When I was diagnosed with breast cancer in 2016 losing my hair was one of the few things I felt like I knew how to rectify. I became quite obsessed with researching the best wigs and having one sitting ready on my dressing table for when my straggly locks made their departure. I remember my cancer nurse telling me there was no rush as it would take at least ten days for my hair follicles to give up the ghost after my first round of chemo, but I was determined that I needed my wig to be ready and waiting weeks before my treatment began.

The thought of losing my hair was keeping me awake at night, I felt quite suffocated by it. At this point I was still very self-conscious and vulnerable about my cancer diagnosis. During another stressed-out night where sleep would not come to let me escape, I came up with a plan to turn this terribly negative situation into a positive one.

So, on 27 July, only 11 days after my first chemo, I shaved my head for charity. I had planned on doing it a few days later but my hair had started to fall out and I just wanted it gone. I had begun to hate touching my hair and even looking at it. Shaving my head was the best thing I could have done; instead of weeping over my ever-decreasing mop, I – and my husband, in a true act of solidarity – shaved our heads in my living room, with smiles on our faces, and raised over £3,000 for the Beatson Hospital, where I was having my treatment.

This was a huge turning point for me in my attitude to having cancer. It gave me a complete confidence boost. If I could shave my hair off and walk around for all to see, I could do just about anything. After the head-shave my Instagram and blog @cancerwithasmile really took off, and I grew in self-belief and got strength from sharing my story with cancer fighters all over the world.

Strangely, what actually hit me harder than chopping my mop was when the little spikes that remained jumped ship too and I was left with a shiny dome. The sad feelings didn't last long and soon my kids, husband and I were well used to my lack of hair.

Now we come back to that gorgeous wig I was so hell-bent on having ready. As it turned out, Barbie (my creative name for my long blonde wig) and I did not build a lasting relationship. I'm a bit of a fusspot when it comes to certain fabrics on my skin. Wool and I do not get on well, so wearing a wig was just not for me. I decided my head covering of choice would instead be pretty scarves. I just found them so much more comfortable and less fuss. I invested in a little collection so I could change things up and watched a few YouTube videos to learn different ways to tie them. New Look is where I got most of mine and they were a bargain at about six quid each. The best ones to get are square and not too silky or they tend to slide off, although I did discover that spraying silky numbers with a bit of starch spray and giving them an iron helped give them a bit more structure. For days when I was in a right rush or didn't even have the energy to tie scarves, cotton beanie hats from eBay saved the day. I got a funky selection of different colours with star-shaped studs on them for around £5 a go. All in all, losing my hair was not nearly as bad as I expected and I now sport a bleached pixie do, which I love but never would have had the guts to try pre-cancer, so silver linings and all that.

To Wig or Not to Wig?

Wigs: My experience of wig shopping broke me. I did some research and went to a variety of places, some 'off the peg' lower-cost and some bespoke options that you would need to remortgage to afford. You will be informed by your nurses whether or not your treatment plan includes drugs that will mean you are likely to lose your hair. If you know you will lose your hair and want to wear a wig, go shopping before your treatment starts. The best wig-makers have lists stretching into next year, and just ordering a decent one to fit you can take a while.

Take a friend with you if you can – I found the whole experience overwhelming and I didn't really take in much of what was being said because all I could think about was if my lopsided head would look weird without hair! Shop around – find a place you feel comfortable in. I had some bad experiences when staff didn't quite seem to understand what an emotionally big deal this whole thing was for me; there was no way they'd have got my hard-earned pennies, no matter how desperate I was for new locks!

Headscarves: If headscarves are more your thing, go for it. Be bold and try out different styles. YouTube is full of 101 ways to tie a headscarf.

Hair Replacement Systems: They are expensive, but if I had lost my hair I was going to opt for a 'system'. It's a semi-permanent hairpiece that is woven into any existing hair, and means you don't wake up bald, which was my main fear! It's not suitable for everyone and maintenance is expensive too, but for me that investment would have been worth it. Do some research and shop around for those with good reviews.

Warning: People focus on losing their head hair, but your eyebrows and lashes might go too! There are some excellent options such as micro-blading and 3D stick-on pieces, but you need to be aware of how your skin will react. When my eyelashes started falling out I got some extensions put in. For one day, I proudly declared they were the best thing

EVER, until while sitting at a posh dinner the next evening they started falling into my soup one by one... It turns out not all beauty treatments are suitable while you're on chemo!

Using the Cold Cap

I've mentioned this before. Think of it as a modern torture method that if you grit your teeth enough you will get through. Is it worth it – absolutely. Is it for everyone? Absolutely not! Depending upon your regime, you may be offered the use of a cold cap to help reduce hair loss. It does just what it says on the tin – it's a cold hat, soooo cold in fact that you will have ice in your hair upon removing it. If you can get through the first ten minutes, though, your head goes numb and the rest is plain sailing! I tried juggling, plate-spinning, dancing, marching and word repetition to get through the initial pain. And it worked! I know I've said I didn't lose my hair, but it did thin – but without a shadow of a doubt, in the cycles I wore the cold cap, the thinning was significantly less. So I say give it a go and then decide how you feel; you may be surprised at how easily you cope with it. (Or not!)

Ensure the cold cap fits like a glove to get the maximum effect – be really particular about this (your nurse will guide you) and play around with different sizes until it hugs your head properly.

In summary:

- Look after the hair you have. Limit washing it to twice per week and generally be gentle on it; you don't have to stop brushing it, but hold the roots when you do. Buy gentle shampoo that is as chemical-free as possible.
- Be kind to your scalp and nurture it – healthy hair growth comes from a healthy scalp.
- If you keep your hair and you usually go, or start going, to a salon, get blow-dries and add in deep-conditioning treatments. This will not only make you look and feel good but will also help condition your existing hair.
- If your hair falls out, looking at the clumps may feel worse than looking at your reflection. So don't look at it. Get out of the shower and ask a friend or relative to bin the evidence.

- Go wig shopping before you start treatment and shop around for the best options for you.
- Try out the cold cap; it really helps reduce hair loss. And it's an experience in itself – give it a go, even just to give your chemo buddy a laugh and a half.
- It's not 'just hair' and it's okay to feel scared and sad at losing it. You are not being vain – you are being human!

Did you know that Toni and Guy have teamed up with Macmillan Cancer Support to offer a service for anyone whose hair has been affected by chemotherapy? It's called 'Strength in style' and they can advise on hair thinning, hair loss and wig styling. Contact your local Toni and Guy salon for more details.

Love Your Scars – From Baggy Jumpers to Naked Shoots!

Beauty is not about being a perfect cover girl with no imperfections. In fact, the more photoshoots I find myself at, the more I realise that clever lighting can work wonders, and that most images we perceive as desirable are heavily Photoshopped. I'm amazed at how much 'hotter' the edited version of me is!

I've always been quite confident in myself. I use clothes and make-up to feel sexy, and exercise makes me feel strong. When single, I'd be the first to just shamelessly bee-line for a hot guy in a bar, without any fear of rejection, believing it was their loss anyway if they weren't interested.

I was therefore shocked at how much the scars I gathered from my various cancer-related operations affected my body image and confidence. While I didn't lose my hair, I did lose my ability to feel sexy and feminine. I'd stare at my fresh scars for hours and focus on how 'imperfect' they made me feel in comparison to the perfectly unscarred tummies in the fashion magazines.

And then I met Sophie Mayanne, a wonderful photographer who was putting together a project called Behind the Scars, celebrating both scars and the stories behind them. As I nervously turned up to my first shoot, I was instantly put at ease. I met a variety of inspirational people with a whole host of body scars and I could actually feel myself standing taller as I listened to each one of them. They were so inspiring as they told me the stories behind their scars, how they loved what they represented, their uniqueness and how they were proud of what their bodies had been through. Sophie took some wonderful unedited shots of me, and for the first time I saw I could be sexy and desirable. She has since been documenting my treatment through a series of photographs, even while I've been attached to a chemo pump! I have definitely changed, but over time I've realised that it wasn't my body changing or my scars disappearing, but my growing confidence in what I saw – the smile had come back and the 'this is me and I like it' attitude was once more out in full force!

If you are fresh out of the operating theatre, looking at your scars right now, do you like what you see? If you don't, I promise you it's going to get better. Think to yourself:

- I'm proud of what my body has been through.
- I am sexy.
- These scars make me unique and I love them.
- They are keeping me alive.

I had to work on flipping my mindset so I could look at my body in a different way, but it took someone else capturing me in a light I didn't normally see myself in to really achieve this. It's going to take a while, but before you know it, maybe you'll be throwing caution to the wind and proudly showing off your scars at a photoshoot!

I suggest we aim to carry our scars with pride, knowing they have built us and not defined us.

Make Sure Your Inner Beauty Shines

Cheesy line alert – remember, beauty is in the eye of the beholder. You don't have to look like the new wave of Victoria's Secret models to be beautiful. Beauty and looking 'good' is about having an inner confidence that shouts 'this is me and I'm damn proud of it.' It's about celebrating the beauty behind our scars, our quirks, our uniqueness. But be prepared – it might not come naturally. Cancer treatment will knock your confidence on a variety of levels, so it's not vain to arm yourself with whatever are your favourite tools (a new dress, painted nails, nice perfume) and take some time for you, to boost yourself back up again. Hell, being alive is a big enough excuse to 'dress for the occasion' and if you want to wear sequins on a Monday then do it with pride! Looking good does make you feel better, so slap on some lipstick, because cancer – we're coming to get you!

Looking Good and Feeling Better

TAKE-AWAY TOP TIPS

Here are the 'take-away' nuggets from this chapter to help you feel prepared to face the day and all it may present:

Tip 1 Never underestimate how much better looking good (however you define good) will make you feel.

Tip 2 Your skin, nails and body will change. Invest in good-quality products to help reduce the effects.

Tip 3 Get a good plan of action in place asap if you are likely to experience hair loss. Remember that you have to do what feels right for you.

Tip 4 Know that scars are simply a mark of how strong you are. Learn to love them.

Tip 5 Dress for the occasion and let your inner beauty shine.

• • •

'If you are sad – add more lipstick and attack.'

Coco Chanel

Chapter 8

F*** You Cancer

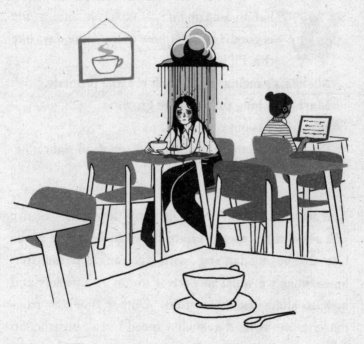

Mental Well-being

What an amazing day it is, sun is shining, life is good. I wonder how many more days like this I'll see?

My heart's racing, and I can't breathe properly.

Maybe my lung tumours are growing.

My cancer is out of control.

I'm so scared that I'm about to drop dead right now.

Fuck you cancer.

Fuck you thoughts.

And welcome to my mind. Is yours like this – or are you as calm as a swan? I have spent the best part of the last 20 years dancing with the anxiety monster. Sometimes we waltz in perfect union and understand how to share the dance floor – other times he frog-marches me around at such a speed I can't breathe. So what's my fear? What fuels my anxiety? What keeps me awake at night?

My fear is the one none of us like to drill down into. But I suspect it's the one we all share to some degree. The one we rarely like to say out loud. Yes – 'I'm scared of dying.' I'm scared that one day, everything I know and love in this world will end. I'm not stupid; I know this will happen for all of us – but, not meaning to be selfish, I want my fair run at life. I want my fair share of time, of laughter, of love – and I'm sure you do too.

In my 'before cancer' life, my fear manifested itself as panic attacks that would strike out of the blue and leave me avoiding elements of daily life. I had a fear of being blindsided by a catastrophic event. Like most of us, I'd experienced a few of those moments where, after a short phone call, life as you knew it flipped. Time cruelly cut short for loved ones, or moments where you feel as though the ground has been whipped from beneath your feet. Rather than it giving me the momentum to live every day, it made me fearful that today might be the day everything changed. The panic attacks that arose would render me frozen in the middle of a busy street. Or make me run out of shop changing rooms half-dressed just because I needed to breathe. Or land me in hospital with a suspected heart attack.

With a lot of help, I got to the point where anxiety was an accepted part of me and through cognitive behaviour therapy, I learned to recognise my triggers and rationalise them before they got out of hand. It wasn't foolproof but it was helpful. And then my biggest fear was realised – I got my diagnosis. No mind games, no overactive imagination, no made-up scenarios – this was my reality.

If right now you have days of blind panic, nights of lying awake imagining the worst, manic highs, crazy lows and everything in between – you are not alone. There is all too often an assumption that dealing with cancer is just a physical problem. That the battle is getting through the chemotherapy, the surgeries, the treatment. But the 'mental' challenge that awaits is even harder. You will be guided through the physical side, step by step, and given hundreds of pieces of information warning you about which side effects you might experience. But they don't warn you about how your emotions will drag you around into a hundred different places, how you will have to learn to carry the dark dog of fear around with you and find a way to function despite knowing what might be round the corner.

I don't have it cracked – I don't think anyone does. But I hope that, by sharing how I deal (or not!) with the rollercoaster, I might be able to give you some comfort and help you to know that EVERYTHING you are experiencing is normal.

It's Okay Not To Be Okay

Have you cracked your 'I'm okay' smile yet? You'll find it will come out just so you don't need to go into details about how you are not actually okay. In fact, you may not be so okay – 30 minutes ago you were sobbing uncontrollably on the kitchen floor, but then you wiped your tears and went to collect the children. I've always thought of myself as pretty hardcore. Despite my over-active mind, I was unflappable when taking on a tough challenge, or under time pressure. I just rolled my sleeves up and got on with it. Chemo – I see you, I've got you. Or so I thought.

And to be fair I did, for most of it. But there are moments when it got me – and that's okay. I had just completed a full chemo regime, and then as my cancer spread and the goalposts started moving, had to start all over again! By cycle 20, things had started to take their toll. My nose was bleeding just from breathing in the cold air, I sounded as if I was housing a mucus production factory and to top it off norovirus had set up a permanent home in my bowels. When your ability to look after yourself regresses to that of a three-year-old, you curl up in a ball and hide under the bedcovers in the hope that food will magically appear in front of you. And you wish for that same magic fairy to dunk you in a bath to get rid of that 'been in bed three days' stench. So, I moved back into my parents', and became my 14-year-old self again. I regressed and cried. I lost half my insides down the toilet. My dad had to hold my hair back as I vomited while also pissing myself (something that hadn't happened to me since I was 18 and overdid it on the party scene). For the first time in a year, I asked to postpone my chemo. I realised I wasn't okay. I felt like shit, I felt beaten and defeated. My body was at breaking point, and I wondered if this was where I should say 'enough is enough.'

'Be kind to yourself,' a wise friend kept saying to me. I had never got this, but now I started to unpick what she was trying to tell me. And I share it with you because it's the best advice I've been given. My feelings were normal, more than normal, and so are yours. I felt frustrated, shattered and I just wanted to sleep. Perhaps, like me, you are annoyed that your body isn't working properly. That this doesn't feel like a 'full life' right now.

'But how can you expect to be okay?' she said. 'You are not a superhuman'. For those of us who like to think everything is fine and to 'keep calm and carry on', lowering expectations may be a hard pill to swallow. But, as I did, you have to learn to be kind to yourself. To know it's okay not to be okay. To stop having a go at yourself or feeling frustrated for not being on top form. You are doing the best you can right now so if you feel like crap let yourself feel like crap!

Coping With the Mental Rollercoaster

Are you prepared for the ride? You will wake up on some days and feel desperate to work through your entire bucket list, while other days will require a fork-lift truck to lift you out of bed. Emotions, for any of us, aren't a pick 'n' mix sweet stand we can choose from each morning. They're much more likely to be a lucky dip.

> **Warning:** You may sometimes find that what are supposed to be the happiest of occasions are ruined by the wave of emotions you simply can't control. But think about it this way – it's ridiculous to look at your diary and think, right life, 11 March tomorrow – I'll wake up feeling happy; cancer thoughts will disappear and all will be well! So if you find yourself sobbing on Mother's Day, party-ing through Easter and not wanting to get out of bed for your birthday – it's ok – shit happens, and you are dealing with a whole ton of it right now – so go easy on yourself.

Do you sometimes feel as if your mind is like a big pair of scales? Perhaps some of these sayings are familiar?

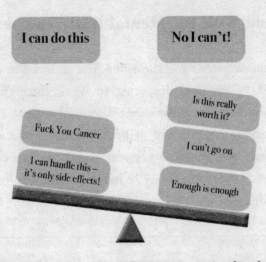

Positive vs negative thoughts

You may spend your day flipping between 'I've got this' and 'no I don't!' So let's look at making the ride smoother. Be prepared for a constant mind battle between feeling like your cheering squad is carrying you and needing to be physically dragged to another chemotherapy or treatment session. Yes, that has happened to me!

I mentioned John back in Chapter 4. He is a 'long-timer' who I met at the Marsden. Twenty years ago he was told he had six weeks to live, but he's still here, just to prove the critics wrong. I chat often to him. On one occasion I was having a really bad day and was beside myself, saying I couldn't do this any more. 'I bet it gets easier,' I said to him. 'Don't you just get used to this?' 'Well actually, no,' said John, who has done over 100 chemo cycles. He told me that it was perfectly normal at any stage to have periods where it all gets a bit too much and you just feel like you need a break – you want to run away and be done with it. Even 20 years on, he said, every five months or so he'd dip, question his treatment, question if it was worth it, get angry, throw his toys out of the pram. He'd then sit down and for three days write down hour by hour the good things and the bad things. His list was always longer on the good side and he would realise it maybe wasn't as bad as he'd thought. He told me that as long as the list was longer on the positives, he'd carry on, just getting on with it. So I did the same, and it worked! It got me mentally to my next chemo cycle; and I still use the strategy now whenever I'm feeling sorry for myself.

If you are stuck in a 'pit' and feel you can't go on, break your day down. Write a list of all the positives and another list of the negatives. Do this for three days. You may realise it's not as bad as you think. If it is, then you MUST speak to friends, family, a doctor or your healthcare team for help right away. It's normal that you might be finding things hard while undergoing treatment, but speaking to someone can be the first step to ensuring you get the support you need. There are free helplines if you are feeling down or desperate – some are open 24 hours per day.

Coping Mechanisms

How do you remain so positive, people ask me. Well it's just wine, I flippantly reply as they laugh and my inner self questions whether lunchtime drinking every day is really acceptable... It's normal that people will turn to a variety of coping mechanisms to get them through treatment. The key is to look for those that are deemed 'negative' and exchange them for 'positive' ones. How many from this list do you know you use – and are they mainly positive or negative?

Shopping	Smoking	Writing	Relaxation techniques
Drinking	Over-sleeping	Talking	Taking time out
Lack of boundaries	Promiscuous	Good sleep routine	Keeping involved with activites

Positive and negative coping mechanisms

The first step in flipping and exchanging the way you cope is to recognise what methods you use. The key thing is that even if you recognise some that are not 'healthy', don't be too harsh on yourself. You are only human after all and you are coping with a big deal!

To Hell and Back – Coping With Cancer Depression

I went through a period of depression but I didn't know it. I only know now, when I look back and understand that I was unjustifiably blaming 'cancer' for everything. I was sleeping all the time – not because I was actually tired; I just had no 'drive'. I never saw highs in my mood, I was drinking – a lot – and I was avoiding people. But then I found writing and writing brought me out of the darkness into the light. It was my way of talking about my fears and emotions and making sense of everything in my mind. I found pleasure in helping others through my words and that in itself helped me.

If you are feeling low there is help out there – please take it! I repeat … no one is too big, too hairy or too old to admit they are finding it hard. And once you've admitted that, then you are already on the path to coping better. Your healthcare team will be able to provide you with options ranging from counsellors to cognitive behaviour therapy, to medication, to group talking sessions. Never underestimate the power of exercise in lifting your mood; and the same goes for friends, and a good book.

Don't feel like you are failing if you need medication. In a conversation with some fellow cancer buddies recently I was rather surprised, but comforted, to find out that a lot of people in the group had visited their doctors and were currently taking medication to help ease their anxiety and lift their mood. If you feel you may need to as well, please take that first step by speaking to your GP or healthcare team. There is no shame in admitting you might need some help, and you'd be surprised at just how many people – who you may think to look at would never need antidepressant medication – might just be on it.

> **Remember!** Watch for the signs of depression and talk to a professional if you are experiencing any symptoms that are worrying you. Depression can manifest in many ways including low mood, sleeping too much, avoiding others, difficulty sleeping, feeling empty and numb, restless and agitated, a sense of unreality and finding little pleasure in activities you used to love. However, many of these symptoms are also regular side effects of cancer treatment, so don't automatically assume if you are feeling rubbish one day that you must be depressed.

Take Time Out to Help Yourself

As I've mentioned before, ideally, we'd all be living in my cancer hotel and with the sun always shining and margaritas on tap. I think that would go a long way to lifting anyone's mood! However, back in the real world, taking time out to focus on healing your mind and giving yourself time to think and reflect is just as important as taking time to dress nicely or tend to the garden weeds! Ask yourself these questions:

Do you have a safe space? Your 'go-to' place of Zen? Perhaps it's clutter-free and minimal; perhaps it's cosy – but it's yours and you feel secure there.
Does your home allow you to have time out to yourself? Even if it's just an hour in the bath, do you have a space that you can call your own?
When and where do you feel most relaxed? This may not be at home. What is it about the space that makes you relax? If it's not in your house, can you recreate it at home?
When was the last time you had a change of scenery or routine? Think about taking a holiday if the pennies allow, or a weekend away or day trip to the countryside, or how about the sea?
What items on your list can others do for you? Remember that people are generally only too happy to give you some help – don't feel worried about asking for it.

Face Your Biggest Fear

Do you want to talk about what happens if things don't work out, but no one around you wants to engage? I wanted to chat all things morbid. I wanted to discuss where my funeral would take place, where my ashes would be scattered (Kew Gardens and Richmond Park, of course!) and how the kids would get dressed in the morning without me. I wanted to ensure that if I died someone would still take my daughter shopping for tacky goods and cuddle my son if he hurt himself. The more I wanted to talk, the more people would tell me to stop talking like that – it scared them. They weren't ready to face what might be, but it made me frustrated because I wanted and needed to talk. I took myself to see a counsellor and I'd highly recommend you do the same. There are many counselling services connected to hospitals, so ask your healthcare team for a referral.

While it's not good for lifting that mood to talk about your mortality every day, it is important to discuss it with friends, family or a specialist counsellor if you feel it will help you. You also need to be realistic with where you are in your journey and if it is in fact a very real possibility or just you jumping to the worst-case scenario. You need to explain to those close to you how it will help you deal with your diagnosis and then ring-fence dedicated time to get things off your chest. Say it as many times as you need to, but then don't dwell – move on.

Positive Mindset – I Can, I Will, I Am – Fuck You Cancer

I don't think any of us know just how tough we can be until we have to be. People tell me I'm brave, and I'm sure they tell you the same. But I respond by saying 'Well it's not like I have a choice to be anything else!' I consider myself to be resilient – I am an ex-national gymnast and my background of training 30 hours a week, under the watchful eye of coaches who wanted me to be the best of the best, meant that it was drilled into a young Deborah that when you failed you went back and tried again. You persisted until you landed the flip on the beam or you could perform that giant swinging circle on the bars. Giving up mentally was not an option – even when you were shit-scared at the age of ten that you were about to fly off the bars and break your neck! I believe that as a result I have what Carol Dweck calls a 'growth mindset' – which means I believe that success is based on hard work and a positive frame of mind.

Dweck believes that success doesn't derive from pre-set, or innate, intelligence but from an individual's mindset or beliefs about themselves. For example, do you genuinely believe you can get through chemotherapy? In her book *Mindset* Dweck explains there are two views of intelligence and capacity for achievement: the first says it's immutable and you are born that way – a fixed mindset; the second view (the growth mindset view) believes that success is changeable – malleable – we can see failure as a way of bettering ourselves and strive to learn from it.

Let me get this straight – I don't for one second believe I can 'beat' cancer by just being positive, believing that

I will never give up and claiming 'I can change my outcome.' But I do think this approach can be used to help us approach treatment we might be apprehensive about. I have spent years looking at the impact instilling a growth mindset in students can have on learning outcomes. The results can be incredible. A growth mindset can give students who previously believed that they couldn't improve their ability an opportunity to reach for the stars.

I believe we can use this approach to help give us hope even in the darkest of cancer days. If we remove hope from our journey then what are we left with? Are we just succumbing to following the expected path and not believing we may be that lucky person who defies the odds? Do we crumble at each setback or failure, perhaps believing it's our fault? It's not your fault if chemo doesn't work – you just need to look at how to rise up from it and see it as an opportunity to improve both your treatment pathways and your overall quality of life.

What gives me hope, even when I feel that the situation is hopeless, is to look for those miracle stories. We all too often hear of those that don't end well, but do you actively seek out examples of when it has? Go and hunt them out and take inspiration from them. I can't promise it will make things okay, and I can't promise it will rid you of cancer, but I would much rather live with hope – and I'm sure you would as well.

Can a 'Growth Mindset' Help?

'Stop crying – you have to be positive to beat cancer!' 'You can do this!' Well, if beating cancer was that easy do you not think we'd all be given anti-crying medication, happy pills and a motivational trainer? I appreciate I've just waxed lyrical about how great having a positive attitude is – but is there any evidence that it will help us live longer with the big C? I wish that positivity did work – but sadly to date there is no robust evidence from studies to show that a positive mindset prolongs cancer survival after diagnosis. In fact, despite many large-scale studies, including one that followed 60,000 people for 30 years, there is still no known link between personality type (positive or not) and higher risk of cancer. So, looking at it from the other side, being grumpy for a day is NOT going to make your cancer grow! I think it's fair to point out here that you should not feel pushed into being 'positive' and upbeat if that's simply not going to work for you. Never feel guilty about your mood having an impact on your cancer spreading – it won't and please don't listen to anyone who tries to tell you otherwise!

So does trying to keep a positive mindset have any part to play? In the last few decades research HAS shown that having a positive mindset can reduce tension, anxiety and tiredness and reduce the risk of depression in cancer patients. A recent report also states that this then leads to fewer hospital admissions than among those who suffer from these conditions.

But I think it's important that we look beyond the data here and ask – well, does it make me FEEL better? For me the key thing is how to be as 'normal' as possible while living with cancer. It's about feeling good in the time we have and using our mind in a positive way to help us deal with all that is thrown at us.

My friend Brenda Trenowden is a fabulous example of someone who is determined just to roll her sleeves up and still run an international organisation while having chemotherapy! Okay, we can't all be as hardcore as Brenda, but I think we can take a lot from her positive 'I can do this' approach:

> I'm a reasonably fit and healthy person and I'm very active – I have a fairly demanding day job as a banker, I lead a global campaign called the 30% Club aimed at achieving better gender balance in senior leadership roles, I have a lovely family and

lots of friends and I try to make time for running as well. In fact, I was feeling so fit and well that I took up the offer of a routine health check at work, to have my health validated. It was and I passed with flying colours – at 49 years of age, I was in the best shape I've been in for years. However, I did have a distended tummy, which I assumed was due to age, having two children and having had a C-section.

At the end of the exam, the doctor suggested a smear test and internal exam as well. She noted that my uterus was slightly enlarged and suggested I follow up with an ultrasound. I did so and was very surprised when the results showed a large mass and fluid, which led to CT scans and a consultation with an oncologist gynaecologist. I didn't allow myself to worry – with my 'glass half full' attitude, I assumed it would be fibroids or something benign.

I can remember the moment I got the news very clearly. It was a few weeks later and I was in a meeting in the City when my phone rang.

I did have cancer; it was a very rare one-in-a-million type of appendix cancer called pseudomyxoma peritonei. The oncologist told me that that there are not many places in the world that specialise in it as it's so rare, but that one of the centres of excellence is in Basingstoke and he was going to write to the surgeon there and ask him to see me.

I was stunned. Walking to London Bridge to get the train home, I felt as though I was in a bubble. I was looking at everyone thinking you don't know how lucky you are to be normal. I felt like I was a different species on a foreign planet. I was one of those people with cancer. I couldn't quite process the information.

My husband and I spent that weekend googling it, which was a mistake. One article referred to it as a 'doozy' and the author said 'if you get it, you're in trouble ... Of all the cancers I'd like to never have (all of them) this one comes somewhere near the top of the list.' Not what I needed to hear.

However, the following week when I got to meet the surgeon, I felt happy and reassured – he had done 700–800 surgeries and was one of the best. He explained the surgery and that recovery would take about four months and be hard, but said that he thought he could cure me. We scheduled surgery for the fourth of January so that I could enjoy Christmas with the family and he told me to keep up my fitness as it would help with my recovery. I actually left feeling very positive and lucky – lucky that it had been found, lucky that I was being treated by one of the top surgeons in this rare disease, lucky that the clinic was in the UK and only two hours from home and lucky that I had a chance at a cure.

My wonderful running buddy agreed to 5:30am runs (with headlamps) in the park near my home up until the surgery and I had a lovely Christmas. I didn't think about the surgery or what was coming afterwards. I just spent time enjoying life, family and friends. Somehow, I was able to compartmentalise it.

The practical side of me did kick in and I spent time going through my life insurance and other financials and produced spreadsheets for my husband, Trend, outlining how the family would survive if I died in surgery. Trend hated it, but it made me feel better to have done it. What I didn't tell him was that I had kept all of the receipts from the clothes, shoes and other things that I had bought in the post-Christmas sales, so that he could return them if I didn't survive. Once again, being practical made me feel in control. The other thing that I needed to sort out was a communication strategy. I have a large network of friends around the globe and I was conscious that they would all be ringing the house and wondering how I was doing. I didn't want Trend having to go through this time and time again, so I set up a site – www.brendawontbackdown.com. I wrote a few blogposts about how I was feeling having been diagnosed, which was really cathartic for me, and then from the day of the surgery Trend took over. It was brilliant. We had so many supportive and lovely comments, which he read to me in hospital. They really helped fuel my resilience. It was also good for Trend as he enjoyed writing the updates and getting the feedback without having to take lots of calls.

The surgery was as horrific as I'd been warned, and they took out my appendix, gall bladder, spleen, uterus, ovaries, part of my bowel and the outer lining of my liver. I woke up the day after happy to be alive and managed to go home after only two weeks. Although my company was very supportive and told me to take as long as I needed, I was back part-time after four months, and very quickly got back up to full-time with two days a week working from home. I didn't need to have time off, I needed to get back to normal – both in my day job and in my campaigning and meeting with people for the 30% Club. I think that really helped my resilience – a strong sense of purpose and control and a very supportive family and network of friends. I also felt very strongly that I didn't want people to write me off because I had had cancer.

I quickly turned my mind to my career and how to move on to the next phase. With my fiftieth birthday on the horizon, I thought I should work towards promotion to the next exec position. Once again an unexpected event turned things upside down for me (this cancer thing was getting very inconvenient and messing up my plans!).

I had a scan ten months after the surgery and found that the cancer had come back. I was referred to an oncologist, had a port-a-cath fitted and started a six-month programme of 12 chemo sessions just before Christmas,

Once again, our Christmas had cancer running along in the background; and once again, I was determined to keep up with all of my activities and not let this get in the way. I have managed to only take every other Wednesday off work for the chemo and then either go into the office with my chemo pump in a nice cross-body bag, or work from home the following two days depending on the weather (as one of the side effects is a bad reaction to the cold).

I decided that rather than dread the chemo, I would find a way to look forward to it. So every other Wednesday is a 'Chemo Salon' where lots of friends come round with soup and bread. We all have a brilliant time, take fun selfies and I don't even notice the poison flowing into my veins. It's brilliant. I've caught up with friends I haven't seen in years.

Obviously the chemo is not nice; the side effects are a pain in the ass and the fact that I am likely to need more surgery at some point down the road and further chemo to manage this chronic condition is not great. But somehow I can't feel sad or bitter about it. I love my life and this cancer experience has had many upsides.

Most importantly, facing my own mortality has really forced me to be focused on leading a very purposeful life, spending time with people I want to be with, doing all the things I had put off (theatre, concerts, travel, visiting friends and family) and saying what I want to say to people. I'm very happy and fulfilled and I am determined to beat this beast or at least tame it.

F*** You Cancer!

TAKE-AWAY TOP TIPS

Here are the 'take-away' nuggets from this chapter to help you navigate the mental rollercoaster that comes alongside your diagnosis:

Tip 1 Have an initial plan and know it may change – accept that this is part of living with cancer.

Tip 2 A growth mindset may not change your prognosis but it can change your quality of life.

Tip 3 Ask for and accept help from professionals to help you cope with the mental stress of cancer.

Tip 4 It's okay not to be okay – but try to brush it off and see what tomorrow holds.

Tip 5 Always have hope, even in the darkest days.

• • •

'Always believe that something wonderful is about to happen.'

Dr Sukhraj Dhillon

Chapter 9

Mashed Potato and Red Wine: A Healthy Lifestyle and A Happy Balance

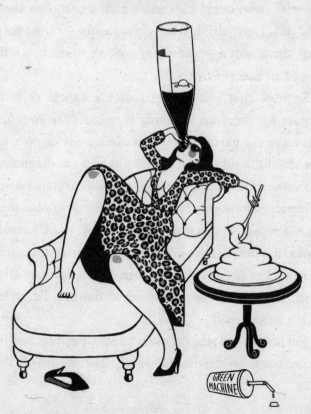

Food That's Fit For You: Green Juice, Turmeric and McDonald's

Have you tried turmeric? I knew a guy once who cured his cancer with wheatgrass shots. Don't drink wine, drink coffee – oh no sorry don't drink coffee – and sugar – don't touch it, it's the root of all cancer evil!

So now that you are part of the cancer club, be prepare for everyone believing they can cure you! You will receive a barrage of well-meaning advice on what you should/shouldn't eat as soon as you are diagnosed, and some kind friends might go as far as to start weekly deliveries of food only fit for a rabbit hutch to your front door. I'm not exaggerating when I tell you I have 16 books that people have given me about eating for cancer patients; I've realised that if I were to amalgamate all of them, and then throw in my vegetarianism, I'd be left with a lettuce leaf!

I'm not here to slag off every cancer-busting, healthy eating book or activist. However, let's not forget that

I'm the ex-gymnast vegetarian who still got bowel cancer. So if anyone has grounds to be a little sceptical about those advocating that a raw food diet is the source of all cancer cures – it's me! But I am all about balance and letting your body tell you what it needs. We need to understand what the research is really saying we should and shouldn't eat, and how that might affect the choices we make, and of course as a strict vegetarian of 25 years, how can I not advocate the benefits of a healthy eating plan? I don't choose a salad because I think it will cure me of cancer; I choose it because it makes me feel good. I enjoy understanding the impact food can have on my mood and energy levels and how my body just feels better when it's fuelled well. I eat for enjoyment and I hope that I make choices that will, in turn, help keep my immune system strong enough to handle all the toxic concoctions and surgery that is thrown at it.

But I Just Want McDonald's!

Let's be very clear that while you are undergoing treatment, and especially if you are on chemotherapy, anything goes. And by anything I mean you have total free rein to tell the well-meaning green-juice-drinking campaigners to go do one (if that's what you want). If you want to eat McDonald's for three days in a row for breakfast, lunch and dinner then that is exactly what you should do. I did (yes it was the veggie version!) – and it got me through another chemo cycle without vomiting. Chemo, as I have described in Chapter 3, can have a barrage of stomach-related side effects – that may mean your stomach churns at the sight of food or you vomit at the smell of cheese. Your weight may plummet and the lack of nutrients make you feel weak. Your immune system needs to be in the best state possible to accept and tolerate chemotherapy and the odd lettuce leaf and a splattering of chocolate won't place you in the best position. I've overheard many conversations on the chemo ward between nurses and other patients whose weight is plummeting – 'Have you tried milkshakes and Mars Bars?' If these experts are so relaxed about patients eating these, then obviously this is not the time for you to worry about calorie-counting! It's just about getting food inside you that will give you strength – and, most importantly, that you can keep down. People have all too often steered me in the direction of a barrage of vegetable juices and smoothies. Try pouring only vegetables into a newly resected bowel and not having to leg it to the loo at 100mph! What I really needed was hardcore stodge like potatoes and rice.

Your Body Knows

I will never forget my recovery after my bowel resection. This was when my clever surgeon, essentially, took out the tumour and put my bowel back together. Recovery from this operation is tough because everyone is waiting with bated breath for you to pass your first fart – this is a celebration in itself because it means your bowel has woken up again – and a poo, well that's just cause for a full-on dance festival! But after I'd had three days on a liquid diet, producing poos like a baby's, my surgeon entered my room to find me, having had no sleep, sobbing and shattered by not being able to tell the difference between gas and a 'follow-through' – and with a stomach that was fed up with jelly! What's wrong, he calmly asked. 'Well, I just want my own bed, for starters – and then I really just want mashed potato and some red wine,' I proclaimed. He promptly discharged me and that night I got my bed and I got mashed potato and my bowel was happy. So happy in fact that my first solid poo followed, which was call for a ball! A poo party that thankfully included the red wine I also craved. My body knew, and yours might just know too – so listen to it.

Help Me!

When you have a stomach that feels like it's on a constant rollercoaster, what practical things can you do to help?

- Aim for 6–8 small meals per day rather than three large ones. Aim to eat every 2.5 hours throughout the day.

- Smoothies are lifesavers. Get yourself an easy-to-clean blender or juicer. Yes, I take the mickey out of the juicing brigade, but I love red berry smoothies and I'm sure they helped give me energy during my chemo. When you just don't feel like eating, try a little yogurt, banana, honey and raspberries in the blender and before you know it, you'll have consumed some of your daily calorie intake – and kept it down!

- Whatever you ate in hospital during your chemo sessions, you may struggle to eat once you're back home because of the associations or the sheer repetition. So stick with the same meal each time you are in hospital, and just recognise that you may not be cooking it at home any time soon! For me, each chemo cycle I had jacket potato with cheese and beans. It's safe to say I haven't eaten this since.

- Chemo mouth is a real thing! Everything may taste a little funny, but fizzy water will, on the whole, taste acceptable. Your mouth will thank you for the cleansing feeling.

- Always have boiled sweets to hand. Mints and fruit-flavoured sweets can do wonders to settle an icky tummy and lubricate a dry mouth.

- Internet shopping, especially for your groceries, is your new best friend. Sign up and get the basics delivered once or twice each week.

- Consider 'cook at home' delivery services. There are many companies that deliver the ingredients for healthy, home-cooked food, ready for you or your partner to whip up following a recipe card. They aren't the cheapest option, certainly not for every day, but I really enjoy attempting (and I do mean attempting) to cook a meal when I haven't used up all my energy shopping for the ingredients. I tend to buy in three meals for two people per week, which keeps the cost down a bit.

- Have two or three easy-to-create snacks in your fridge always. When you are tired it's easy to forget about, or not be able to face, making food, unless it's super-easy. It's very reassuring knowing that your snacks are there, and that it takes two minutes to put them together. Each week during chemo, I always made sure I had my preferred ingredients in the house. My go-to, two-minute list is below – what's yours?
  - Cottage cheese with pineapple on Ryvita.
  - Greek yogurt, honey and banana.
  - Ready-made egg mayo to pop into a sandwich any time.

- A tin of cream of tomato soup – never underestimate the power of tinned soup!
- A bowl of rice crispies (I craved them at any time of day!).
- Hummus and pitta bread.
- Blueberries, raspberries, pineapple, passion fruit, mango, melon – in any combination. All really refreshing in the mouth.
- Cheese, crackers, grapes.

Winner or Loser?

I just assumed that everyone lost weight during chemo. But nope, not me – I actually gained weight and, in fact, many people do. The steroids meant that my appetite was at an all-time high. If you, like I did, find yourself on the midnight steroid munchies train, try to find an option that doesn't include KFC, McDonald's and Nando's all in one day – make sure you have a look at my quick and easy options above. Now, as I've said, is not the time to worry about your weight; however, if you are feeling unhappy about your body image then please speak to your healthcare team who can point you in the direction of some resources to help you. At the back of this book there is a list of key resources that you can also use as a starting point.

Cancer-Proof Me!

What you need to recognise is that there are foods that in research terms have proven 'interesting', but that there is no hard evidence right now to suggest they can CURE cancer. So we can't write them off, but we also can't make claims with any certainty about the impact they have. And you need to recognise that you can't cancer-proof your life! There is evidence that some life-style choices can put you more at risk for particular cancers, but you need to know that following a healthy lifestyle doesn't necessarily protect you from them either. You still must know your body and understand what is normal for you so that any changes you notice can be checked out asap. Early diagnosis is the key to ensuring we all live longer with cancer.

Is Turmeric Really a Superfood?

'You MUST take turmeric supplements,' everyone declares as soon as you even mention the big C word. Turmeric has indeed demonstrated anti-inflammatory and anti-cancer activities in lab studies and, while we need more studies to verify its benefits, current research looks interesting. There are theories that curcuminoids, a substance found in turmeric, may protect the body in a variety of ways.

Turmeric can act as an antioxidant by neutralising free radicals, and in lab rat experiments it has even been shown to stop the replication of tumour cells when applied directly to them. HOWEVER – recent studies have also shown that it might interfere with some chemotherapy drugs used to treat breast cancer. The jury is out on how this clearly powerful food might help cancer patients. So before you jump onto the turmeric train – check with your oncologist if it would be a beneficial supplement for you. For guidance and more information on interactions and cautions, the Memorial Sloan Kettering Cancer Center is excellent – please refer to the resources section.

Vitamins and Herbs

If many of my friends had their way they would have been throwing vitamins into the atmosphere in the hope they'd boost my immune system! But what people quite often fail to recognise is that while you are undergoing treatment not all supplements and immune-boosting super-pills are good for you – in fact, they can have a detrimental effect and stop the chemo doing its magic. The Memorial Sloan Kettering Cancer Center in New York, which I've mentioned above, designed and runs an excellent, highly regarded website resource, fully cross-referenced and based on up-to-date research.

The information can help you determine which herbs, over-the-counter dietary supplements or superfoods might interact badly with your treatment plan and possibly even stop your drugs being as effective as they can be. I highly recommended having a good look at all the information for any supplements you are considering. And always remember to cross-check the information with your healthcare team.

But I Love Wine!

And don't a lot of thirtysomethings? 'Can I still drink wine?' I asked my oncologist as I signed the consent form to my first ever regime – 'Save the expensive stuff until after treatment,' he said. I assumed he meant for celebrating, but no, he meant that taste buds may change and you'll pick up a fetish for cheap nasty wine – it's true that I did! While there are some drugs that do interact badly with alcohol, the majority do not. Choosing to drink is your choice so, first, don't feel guilty if you do choose to continue to enjoy a glass of wine or two. You may find that your stomach will not be able to handle particular drinks you used to enjoy – beer just makes me feel sick now, for example. The key thing, as always, is to drink responsibly and within guidelines. For more information and guidance please visit: www.drinkaware.co.uk.

Keeping Active (Shake Your Arse and Just Dance)

I have always been sporty. At school I was sports captain, and keeping active has always been part of my life – I enjoy it and I believe it's given me an advantage going into treatment. Despite major procedures including four lung operations and a bowel resection, intensive-care stays, collapsed lungs and drains left, right, and centre, on the whole I've been blessed with a quick recovery from every operation. There is no shadow of a doubt that this has been partly down to my overall level of fitness. The key is to maintain a good level of fitness in whatever way works for you. If you love it, you'll most likely stick at it! I love to dance and managed to find a way to still shake my arse even whilst on a chemo pump!

Keeping Active During Treatment

Evidence shows that exercise can offer many benefits. There has been research showing that those who undertook exercise at least four times per week were less likely to be anxious or depressed while going through cancer treatment. Studies also show that exercising can help to reduce treatment-associated fatigue. As tiredness and weakness are recognised as the most common side effects of treatment, it is very positive news that exercise can be used to help combat this. And weight-bearing exercises such as running or dancing may protect bones against thinning; this is particularly significant for women who have hormone-dependent cancers, as for these patients osteoporosis is a major concern.

Researchers have also looked into the safety of exercise while undergoing treatment, and in general recommend the same level of activity for people with cancer as for the general population.

Generally doctors advise at least 30 minutes a day, five days a week, of moderate-paced activity such as walking. This level of activity is helpful for people even during treatment. But everyone is different and exercise needs to be tailored to you, taking into account your overall fitness, diagnosis and other factors that could affect your safety.

Some exercise tips are:

- Build up gradually.
- Some days you will have more energy than others – it won't be a steady increase.
- Even if you are feeling tired, try 30 minutes of gentle walking.
- Join a fitness class – see the resources section; many cancer support organisations can advise on classes specifically targeted at cancer patients.

There is no evidence that yoga can prevent cancer, but there IS evidence that it can help you cope with side effects. Yoga promotes a natural way to help you relax, and while advanced classes can be strenuous, if you do it under proper guidance it is generally considered very safe. A recent study deemed it the most accessible and easy-to-pick-up form of exercise going.

Studies showed that those who practised yoga regularly throughout treatment had improved sleep and reduced tiredness, anxiety and depression in comparison to those who didn't exercise. Do have a look at the published research on yoga, to be found on the Cancer Research UK website, for more information.

Please note: People with certain types of cancer might need to avoid certain exercise. Please speak to your healthcare team for advice, especially if you have cancer affecting your bones, low immunity, peripheral neuropathy or breast cancer (this, for example, would mean you must take any upper-body exercise very slowly and carefully).

Keeping Active After Treatment

So I haven't signed up to the London Marathon yet – but I have dreams to! Just the small problem of getting my lungs to function and the feeling back into my feet to address first... But there is a really good reason why keeping up your activity levels after treatment is important. Studies have shown that up to four out of ten people are depressed after cancer treatment; as we've seen here, exercise can boost your mood and reduce anxiety and depression – so now is the time to get your running trainers or walking boots on!

There are many different types of activities and some hospitals and organisations, such as Maggie's Centres, run a variety of exercise workshops for people undergoing treatment, which can help you decide which ones you might like to get more involved in. Just to get you started, why not try out three things from this grid for 30 minutes each:

Swimming	Tennis	Brisk walking	NHS Couch to 5km App	Pilates
Salsa	Dance aerobics	Cricket	Gentle circuit training	Yoga

If you feel that your level of fitness is low at the moment and you want to improve it, do have a look at the NHS Couch to 5km app (see the back of this book). It is an excellent – and free – resource that guides you, week by week, through training, with the aim of getting you running (at your own pace) a distance of five kilometres.

We Need to Exercise Our Minds Too! (Mindfulness)

In Chapter 8 we looked at how keeping a positive mindset can help us when the dark cloud closes in. Exercising our minds is just as important as feeding ourselves healthy food and exercising our bodies. As well as exploring the positive mindset research discussed in the previous chapter, I cannot recommend enough that you look into mindfulness activities to help you. Mindfulness helps us focus on the moment, to accept our feelings and thoughts without judgement. It helps us to stop feeling bad about feeling sad or down and to accept and understand that there is no right or wrong way to feel at any given time. We can use these techniques to exercise our minds during treatment.

When I was a teacher, we used mindfulness in our school as part of the national programme on mindset. Here are my top three practical mindfulness exercises that we used as part of the in-school programme that you too can use to calm your mind, and help you face the challenges ahead:

The Three-Minute Breathing Space

Unlike meditations or a body scan, this exercise is quick to perform and is an easy way to get started with mindfulness.

In a busy life, keeping a quiet and clear head can be a challenge, and this exercise is a wonderful technique to help with that. The exercise breaks down into three sections, one per minute, and works as follows:

- The first minute is spent on answering the question, 'How am I doing right now?', while focusing on the feelings, thoughts and sensations that arise and trying to give these words and phrases.

- The second minute is spent on keeping the awareness on the breath.

- The last minute is used for an expansion of attention from solely focusing on the breath; feeling how the ins and outs of the breathing affect the rest of the body.

Thoughts often do pop up in the mind. The idea is not to block them, but rather just let them come into the mind and then disappear back out again. Try to just observe them.

Smile in the Mirror

Does that seem ridiculous? It might feel that way when you first practise it (especially if someone walks in on you). But smiling at yourself in the mirror first thing in the morning has many benefits for your well-being. In fact, British research scientists have concluded 'that smiling can be as stimulating as receiving up to £16,000 in cash.' Smiling slows the heart rate and relaxes the body, and it releases endorphins that counteract and diminish stress hormones. It has also been shown to increase productivity in a variety of tasks, which is excellent for making each and every moment of a busy day count.

Mindful Listening

This exercise is designed to open your ears to sound in a non-judgemental way, and more broadly to train your mind to be less swayed by the influence of preconceptions and past experiences. So much of what we 'feel' is influenced by our past – for example, we may dislike a song because it reminds us of a breakup or another period in life when things felt negative. So the idea of this exercise is to listen to some music from a neutral standpoint, with a present awareness that is unhindered by preconception.

Select a piece of music you have never heard before. You may have something in your own collection that you have never listened to, or you might choose to turn the radio dial until something catches your ear.

1. Close your eyes and put on your headphones.

2. Try not to get drawn into judging the music by its genre, title or the artist's name before it has begun. Instead, ignore these labels and neutrally allow yourself to get lost in the journey of sound for the duration of the track.

3. Allow yourself to explore every aspect of the track. Even if the music isn't to your liking at first, try to let go of your dislike and give your awareness full permission to climb inside the track and dance among the sound waves.

4. Explore the music by listening to the dynamics of each instrument. Separate each sound in your mind and analyse each one by one.

5. Home in on the vocals (if it has them): the sound of the voice, its range and tones. If there is more than one voice, separate them out as you did with the instruments in the step above.

The idea is to listen intently, to become fully entwined with the composition without preconception or judgement of the genre, artist, lyrics or instrumentation. Don't think; just hear.

A Healthy Lifestyle and A Happy Balance

TAKE-AWAY TOP TIPS

Here are the 'take-away' nuggets from this chapter to help you focus on a healthy mind and body during your treatment and beyond:

Tip 1   Being healthy is about balance, yes – but while you are going through chemo and feeling sick, eat whatever you like to get you through treatment, build yourself up and thrive in remission – now is not the time to be worrying about that Mars Bar!

Tip 2   Use reliable resources (as listed at the back of this book) to find out what the evidence really is on superfoods and supplements.

Tip 3 Undergoing cancer treatment doesn't always mean you need to slow down, and exercise has lots of proven benefits – so shake that arse!

Tip 4 Exercising your mind is just as important as eating good food and physical exercise.

Chapter 10

From Survivor to Thriver

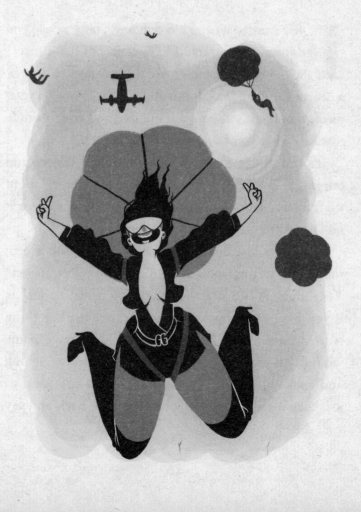

Life 'After' Cancer

If you were to write a bio right now, how would you address your cancer? I have cancer? I had cancer? I'm living with cancer? Are you a cancer patient or a cancer survivor? This is not about what it says on your medical notes; it's about your mindset and your attitude towards what you have been through.

It's not about forgetting you have/had cancer and burying it in a box never to be opened again; it's about using how you look at your cancer and how to turn it into a positive to drive your life forward.

Have you just heard the magic words 'You are in remission?' Congratulations! Can you believe it yet? Yes – there is life 'after' cancer! You probably feel as if you have come back from a war, but the key thing is you have come back! Yes, you may have some wounds to show for it, but you are standing strong and showing cancer who the boss is. Do you want to just take a second to pat yourself on the back and say well done?

You have graduated to a new club – the cancer survivor club – and the good news is that yet again you are not alone! In fact more people are likely to put cancer behind them than not, but now the challenge is becoming a thriver. Adjusting from the mindset of being a cancer survivor to being a cancer thriver won't happen overnight. Just when you thought the tough bit was done, you'll find that more challenges await; but if you can handle the chemo and the operations and the radiotherapy you've already been through – you've definitely got this!

Cancer doesn't just end when your treatment ends. Expect a barrage of emotions and, for some, an onset of shock at what has actually happened and all you've been through. Research indicates that eight weeks after the end of treatment is the most mentally challenging time. By this point you are probably trying to 'move on', and yet the side effects are still present and you are more tired than you ever imagined? Are you trying to rebuild your life and finding it more challenging than you had first expected? Or maybe your 'new eyes' have made you reassess how you want to live your life and you are finding it hard to carve out that new path? For many people it comes as a surprise that you are not just sent on your merry way after treatment with a balloon and a party bag – instead you are back for regular monitoring, blood tests, scans, hormone injections or even maintenance chemo. Alongside these tests comes the big fear of reoccurrence and the mental challenge of allowing yourself to start planning for tomorrow once more. But now is the time to find the right mindset and really start living and recuperating. So where do you begin?

'You Are In Remission'

Just as when you are told 'You have cancer,' when you are told you are in remission your emotions may be all over the place. It actually happened – that goal you have been working towards has actually been met – yes, you've crossed the finish line and you deserve a big fat medal. For me, getting to the point of remission even for a short time was a pipe dream. I was never expecting to get the point of having even one clear scan – so when the words 'Well, your scans are all good' came out of my oncologist's mouth, 16 months after the start of my treatment, I responded with 'Are you kidding me?' What do you mean 'Good' – like no tumours good? I thought to myself. And then I went numb. I had always imagined that if I was ever given the clear-scan news, I'd be jumping for joy, immediately shouting it on social media and popping open the Champagne. Instead, I cried and decided I wanted to hide it from the world.

You may not accept your result at first, pinching yourself and wondering if in fact it was read wrong and something was missed. You may be scared to tell people, as though you might be tempting fate.

As I eventually started to open up about my first clear scan, I delivered the news with a caveat of 'However, we know this won't last for ever' or 'It's just a fluke.' A friend eventually said to me 'Deborah, stop it – change the language you are using. Yes, we know it's probably coming back and yes, that might be in a week, but enjoy this moment.' And she's right – if it does rear its head again, you don't want to regret the worry that clouded the one bright spot you did have.

The Gift that Keeps Giving!

It will come as no surprise to hear that your body doesn't just ping back into a state of normality once what is considered 'active' treatment ends. Cancer recovery is a long road and while you may be done with chemotherapy, operations or radiotherapy for the moment, it's possible and normal that there will be monitoring, medications and treatments still to come. These vary depending on your cancer type, but might consist of, for example, monthly hormone injections and check-ups to monitor longer-term side effects.

Treatment is harsh – fact – and having long-term side effects and changes in the way your body works is totally normal and is a regular part of treatment for many people. How can you expect to pump cytotoxic drugs into your system and for there not to be a backlash! I was really surprised that only after I'd finished chemotherapy did the side effect of neuropathy kick in, meaning that high heels and my numb toes are not a good combination and I have a new-found talent for ripping clothes off due to my inability to undo buttons. This persistent numbness in hands and feet, which I control with a variety of daily creams and patches, has affected my daily life – from the exercise I'm able to do, to having to take more care walking or showering, to having more aches and pains. Mentally it's frustrating. I don't recognise the woman at the back of the gym class who can't touch her toes or who is gasping for breath after five minutes – but then again, I've a friend who says this about herself too and she never had cancer!

Your individual treatment will have a range of more common longer-term complications, and the best advice I can give you is to ensure you get help and ask for referrals to specialists who can work with you to treat and manage them. It's all too easy to assume that just because the cancer has disappeared you no longer need an extra helping hand but, while you may feel you want to be done with seeing the inside of a hospital, burying the symptoms and just muddling on can really impact your quality of life, so address it sooner rather than later.

Don't be alarmed if you end up with an appointment list like when you were first diagnosed! I found myself needing to see so many specialists to help manage side effects that going to the hospital was like a sightseeing tour in itself – from the gastro specialist to talk about my new bowel habits to the hormone people to discuss how mine were acting like a circus and I didn't like their tricks, a lung guy who helps me deal with the side effects that numerous lung operations leave you with and a pain specialist who gives me acupuncture into my nerves to calm the white noise they are firing off into my body – and that's just on a regular Monday visit!

Popping the Cancer Bubble

During active treatment I lived in a cancer bubble. EVERYTHING was cancer. I read cancer, I ate cancer, I generally spent my days being treated for cancer and then worrying about cancer! But this is emotionally draining, and when we are in remission we need to flip that cancer bubble thinking and give it a good pop – we need to get back into the real world.

Start small and start on things that are manageable – routine, food, exercise. Don't start marathon training from day one of being cancer-free (!) but do find a way of exercising that's suitable for you – from dog walking to gardening to cycling. Do it daily wherever possible and increase the amount you do bit by bit. Spend time exploring food and finding things you like to eat. Focus on what makes you feel good, and what you feel fuels your body in a positive way rather than what you feel you 'should' be eating. (See Chapter 9 for more focus on food and exercise.)

Start to set longer-term goals again. Yes, you are in remission, but there are still scans. It may be hard to think of life beyond your next scan – even though it may be a lot further down the line than what you have been used to. But as time goes on, adjust your thinking of your future alongside it. My friends the other day started talking about New Year (in two years' time!) and I freaked! They asked me what I was doing and I instantly responded with 'Well, if I'm alive'... But that needs to change. Start by allowing yourself to book a holiday or an event in advance, a little longer than you are used to doing. This will be different for everyone – I have worked on a 'one month ahead' basis for 16 months, and am currently trying to push myself to two months. Allow yourself to plan what you'd like your life to look like a year in advance – and aim to get to a five-year plan. As we all know, this doesn't mean life will roll like the plan, but it's good for us to allow our minds to go into our future, regardless of what stats may tell us, rather than assuming we don't have a future.

Taking time out from life with cancer is just as important now as it was when you were going through treatment. Take a 'holiday' from cancer: don't allow yourself to Google, read, or talk anything cancer-related for one week. Afterwards, take an hour, sit down and address any 'cancer' thoughts and concerns or 'admin'. Park it and repeat only at fixed times each week, or as infrequently as required. Try to streamline your future cancer admin and do it while at the hospital (waiting rooms can be a productive space for trawling through admin!). It's about trying to compartmentalise your 'cancer life' and your regular life so that it's not all one and the same any more. Cancer has had its fair share of your time up until now, and the less focus it gets from here on in the better!

You Can't Cancer-Proof Your Life – So Live It!

I had a brilliant debate with a very well-known oncologist the other day – but we ended up annoyingly in agreement. I thought he'd be lecturing about how we CAN protect ourselves from the big C, but instead he declared that the more we understand about cancer, the more we learn how genetics are to blame for the vast majority of cancer cases. It is thought that four in ten cancer cases are related to preventable causes, so while there are proven links with diet, exercise and smoking, it's naive to assume that we have the power to prevent all cancers – to, essentially, cancer-proof our lives. I have no proven genetic mutations, don't eat processed meat, or any meat for that matter (which has a link to an increased risk of bowel cancer); I exercise regularly, am not overweight and I don't smoke – and yet I got this cancer that on paper I'm in the lowest risk category for.

So you have a cancer-free window. You may have been thinking – or overthinking – for a while about why you got cancer in the first place. But now try to shift your focus to what can you do to stop it coming back. BALANCE is the key. It's knowing that in the vast majority of cases, there is nothing you did to cause your cancer, and there is not too much you can do to stop it reoccurring. You may see and hear about people who believe the latest super-food cured them, but speak with your healthcare team about what research they believe is relevant for you to look at. I read a case recently about a young man who believed his diet had prevented the reoccurrence of his bowel cancer. However, he shies away from mentioning that he had beforehand had numerous rounds of chemo-therapy, surgeries and 'conventional' treatment, which in the majority of cases cures most people anyway!

So instead it's time to refocus on the big things that we know can give us the strength we need to face the day:

- Get fit and exercise, because it makes you feel strong, gives you energy and releases endorphins.
- Eat well because it fuels your body with energy, and makes you feel healthier.
- Get sleep to allow your body time to relax and recover so you can face the challenge and treats ahead.
- Drink some wine and eat some chocolate – because life is too short!

Dealing With the Fear of the Future

The biggest worry after any clear result is the fear of reoccurrence. Maybe you feel betrayed by your body and are thinking 'Well, if you've tricked me once you'll do it again!' With every tiny niggle, as you have known from the moment the big C came to play, you can no longer just be a regular person who's ill. Are you fearful about getting too comfortable with feeling like life is 'normal' again, only to have it crushed further down the line? Are you worried about finding yourself having to deal with the emotions of being blindsided and your life being thrown up into the air – again? Is it harder because you know that not only are your chances of survival lower if it comes but also that you've had an insight into treatment and you don't like it very much?! These thoughts are very common, and sometimes it helps us just to know that someone else feels the same. Here my friend Emma Campbell shares her thoughts on reoccurrence:

It was the shock that was the hardest part. The blindsiding, hit by a truck, what the fuck, shock. It made no sense. Four years on, four years clear. I was on the cusp of sashaying over the magic five-year mark, celebratory glass in hand, clicking my heels as I crossed the finish line. I was on the cusp of making life for me and my four kids really, really good. I was on the cusp of drawing a line under cancer.

I remember running up the escalators during the rush hour on the way home from work, my fitness levels at a new high thanks to green smoothies, lunges and sit-ups. I remember taking them two at a time, leaving my fellow commuters trailing.

I remember feeling invincible, powerful, strong. I remember feeling like I'd done it, like I'd won.

And then the rash appeared. Gradually at first. A pale-pink, dusky hue that slowly but surely began creeping up over my left breast and up towards my chest.

I decided it was nothing. It must be a reaction to all the exercise I was doing, all the sweat. Or maybe I'd changed my washing powder. Yes, the washing powder, that must be it. Phew.

But I hadn't changed the washing powder and it wasn't the press-ups and planks that were causing my skin to get redder by the day, itchy and hot.

The cancer was back, making its petrifying presence known by changing the appearance of my skin. Later, much further down the line, I would feel grateful that my body gave me clues. That despite me being in tip-top, never-felt-better, shape, I was given a clear sign that something was wrong.

I think one of the most devastating aspects of discovering I was ill again was the realisation that it must have been there all along.

I heard it once and never forgot it – 'If it comes back it means it never went away.'

How could that be?

How could it be that all this time, during the last four years as I recovered and moved forward and picked up the scattered pieces of my broken life and broken body, how could it possibly be that cancer had been there all along? Multiplying, growing, biding its time, cruelly waiting until I was the happiest I'd ever been to strike.

Waiting to take me down.

I thought it was going to do just that. The sky went black. I thought the end had begun. Treatment was brutal, much more so than before. I wept, I protested, I raged from my cosy chemo chair.

'What am I doing here?' I cried to anyone who'd listen. 'I don't understand! I feel so well!'

Do you hear me? I wanted to scream. *I'm well, I'm fine. WHAT AM I DOING HERE?'*

I'M WELL!

But I wasn't well, I was ill.

I had cancer.

Again.

And I really wasn't sure what the future held. I was too scared, still am too scared, to ask.

Staging? I don't know.

Prognosis? I don't know.

Likely survival over the next five, ten years?

I Don't Know.

But I'm doing okay. Better than okay. I'm doing great. Considering. Three years on and life feels normal but not *normal*, normal. It's *cancer* normal. It'll never be completely normal again.

Ongoing treatment every three weeks. 'Maintenance' treatment. Hate that word.

The port pokes up through the thin skin on my chest. My heart pounds as the nurses take vials of blood away to be analysed for signs of raised markers. I shudder. My body shakes and my pulse races as I sit in the waiting room waiting to be called in for the three-monthly appointment with my consultant.

She looks at me as I look at her, frantically reading her face for signs of trouble. Who's going to speak first? Is this the day that I hear that things are going wrong, again?

Is this the day that life falls apart, again?

Is this the day that my luck runs out?

'How have you been, Emma?' she asks, smiling softly, glancing down at my notes.

'Good,' I reply, smiling nervously back. 'Good. Fine. I've been feeling fine. I think I'm fine.'

Am I fine?

And that's life when cancer comes back. When the cancer you thought had gone reveals itself once more.

You think you're fine, you hope you're fine but you just don't know.

But today, as I write, I'm fine.

And that's okay.

I'll take 'fine'.

Fine is good. Fine is bloody great.

www.meandmyfour.com

Instagram: @emplus4

I agree with Emma – fine is okay; in fact fine is aspirational. Fine is the reality of life with metastatic cancer; it's the new normal that you have to accept. But you can still live well with it.

Being a Stage Four-er

For me, a clear scan as a stage four-er is most likely a temporary occurrence, a small window of utter bliss that could last a week, a year – or perhaps, just perhaps, if a miracle occurred, for ever. But I doubt it.

So my clear scan sent me into a tailspin of fear. Fear even darker than when I was first diagnosed. Fear because a dream was realised and yet cancer, when it first came crashing into my world, whipped the floor from underneath me and it might all happen again.

I sometimes feel like saying to people, please don't go around shouting 'I beat cancer' because it makes those who can't or haven't feel like shit. Some of us may never get the chance to shout it from the rooftops – but it doesn't mean we are 'losing'. Cancer hasn't won anything; we haven't lost a battle because we didn't fight hard enough.

In the same sentence that I was told I had a clear scan, I was asked if I wanted to consider maintenance chemotherapy. In my case, a lower dose of chemo for two days every two weeks that, in theory, 'might' keep things at bay for a while longer. 'And how long would this be for?' I innocently asked. 'Well, until it stops working and the cancer comes back' was the response! Oh, so essentially for life. Right.

When someone starts complaining about the six chemotherapy sessions they need, or that the cancer that means they have only an 80 per cent chance of living 20 years is keeping them awake at night, it's all too easy as a 'lifer' to feel anger. You might feel like sitting people down and saying 'Look, I'd kill for that outlook, so get a grip!' Learning not to feel cheated or jealous at other people's diagnosis and celebrations of 'beating' cancer is a difficult but essential pill to swallow. And it's all too easy to forget the challenges that their diagnosis may have brought them – loss of fertility, for example. Cancer at any stage is scary, and you don't have to be at the rubbish end of the statistics to earn the right to have a mental meltdown. Cancer, as we all know, is unpredictable and can surprise us all – in good and bad ways. So make sure you celebrate every small milestone, clear scan or not, and also rejoice in others who do – because any one of us at any moment could have a downturn.

Eyes Wide Open

Cancer made me do it! Many people wax lyrical about the new understanding of the true meaning of life given to them by cancer. And it's true. I don't plan to claim that cancer is the best thing that's happened to me – it's not. But, because of it, I have experienced such raw emotion, had such a hunger to live and experienced a true understanding of what a blessing it is to have life, to be alive, to breathe, to watch my babies grow up – to just smile, laugh and cry. It's heartbreaking that it's taken cancer to make me feel this way and I wish that I could have reached that point without this upheaval. But my 'comfortably numb' life needed shaking up – and maybe yours did too?

So the challenge now is, having finished treatment, do you want to fall back into your old life? If your health allows, will you draw a line under this 'blip' and continue as you always have? Perhaps that life was perfect and you'd love nothing more than to return to it? Or perhaps, like me, you want to question what you will change for the future? There is no better time to re-evaluate and ask yourself a few key questions:

- What do I value most in my life?
- What, if anything, do I regret not doing?
- What do I need to do more of?
- What do I need to do less of?

Thank You

Who has been your guiding light? Who has wiped the tears, provided the wine and swept you up in their arms? Who has got you to stand up and face the day? Who has provided the support, the strength, the laughs? Who did you shout at in your steroid rage, break down in front of and confide in?

While you are undergoing active treatment, it can be harder to recognise what people have done for you. Sometimes, it's fair to say, I was so focused on MY treatment and MY side effects that everything else just faded away. Being in remission gives us time out to reflect on what has gone on and appreciate all the help and support. Say thank you to the people who have been there for you, and make sure they know how much you appreciate what they have done. They have walked with you and will be just as elated as you are at getting to this point. But they, like you, will be affected by the path you've taken together, be shattered by all you have experienced and be scared of what might still come. Hold their hand, wipe their tears for once and tell them you love them. We can't promise to fix each other's problems, but we can promise that we won't ever face them alone.

From Survivor to Thriver

TAKE-AWAY TOP TIPS

Here are the 'take-away' nuggets from this chapter to help you become a cancer thriver:

Tip 1 You have been through a lot – celebrate that you are in remission.

Tip 2 Pop that cancer bubble and start looking to the future again.

Tip 3 Expect side effects and some treatments to continue – but you've done this before and you can do it again!

Tip 4   Don't live in fear of cancer coming back – just live. You can deal with it if it does.

Tip 5   Say thank you to all those who have helped you get to remission and supported you throughout.

• • •

'Surviving is important – thriving is elegant.'

Maya Angelou

F*** You Cancer – Afterword

So as you enter the cancer world, know that as scary as it might be, when you look at others in the hospital waiting room, they too are experiencing what you are. Don't be deceived by those sitting with lipstick on and a smile on their face – inside they are just as worried as you. You will become braver and stronger than you ever thought possible because you have no other choice. You will go through things you never thought you could face – but you will do it, and you will be amazed at how, when tested, you rise to it.

EVERYTHING you are feeling on your emotional rollercoaster is normal, and while I can't guarantee what is round the corner for you, I'm staying firmly with you on the ride, reminding you that you are doing okay – and okay is good – hell, okay is bloody brilliant! I hope I haven't disappointed you by not telling you how to 'beat cancer' – I did warn you at the start that was the case!

All I wanted to do is show you that you are not alone. I'm not the annoying girl who pretends to have her shit together. I stamp my feet, have meltdowns and question how I'm going to get through this on a daily basis – just like you do. I shake when waiting for results, plan my funeral while lying in a CT scanner and overanalyse every one of my oncologist's facial expressions. And this is all perfectly normal.

But I hope that you slip this book into your bag (alongside all that medication you now need to carry, and perhaps that bright lipstick!), and, in those times when you just need an extra bit of reassurance, you flick back and have a read of some of the tips, tricks and reminders I've shared with you. Let's be clear – I don't have the cancer bit cracked AT ALL. I'm leaving that to my fabulous team of specialists, and pray that they CAN crack it. Hell, by the time you are reading this I may not even be here to see the fruits of my labour – and I'd be gutted! But know that these strategies got me to a good point I never believed I'd get to, and they got me through some rough times. I hope they do the same for you. But most of all I pray and hope that you will be able to put cancer behind you some day, and just be you.

If you are up at 3am, just know you have company. I'm lying there wide-eyed too, worrying about what my future holds. I look at my little ones, my loved ones and everything that is wonderful about life and it breaks me to think that it might all end tomorrow. And I know it breaks your heart too. But wipe your tears – for today, writing this, I have life and, reading this, so do you – and for that we are blessed. I may not grow old, but my quality of life will be rich and full of love. And I will know what it means to value every second in life. To feel grateful even when faced with adversity and to make the most out of a bad situation.

Treat life as though it's the most precious thing in the world. For it is. I know that, like me, you will give your cancer a run for its money – a really good run. And maybe, just maybe we'll both be one of the lucky ones. But we have to know that we can't control what these clever little cancer buggers might choose to do, and the less we spend time worrying about that the better. Let's just ensure we enjoy life, laugh a lot, drink the wine, smile in those precious moments, hold those we love close and shout FUCK YOU CANCER as hard as we possibly can, in the hope that it gets the message!

Love Deborah x

Resources

General

Cancer Research UK
www.cancerresearchuk.org

Institute of Cancer Research
www.icr.ac.uk

Macmillan
www.macmillan.org.uk

Maggies
www.maggiescentres.org

Marie Curie Cancer Care
www.mariecurie.org.uk

National Institute for Health and Care Excellence
(NICE)
www.nice.org.uk

NHS – Live Well
www.nhs.uk/live-well

Penny Brohn
www.pennybrohn.org.uk

Stand Up To Cancer
www.standuptocancer.org.uk

American Society of Clinical Oncology
www.asco.org

Memorial Sloan Kettering Cancer Center
www.mskcc.org

Memorial Sloan Kettering Cancer Center – Nomograms
www.mskcc.org/nomograms

Bowel and Other Cancers

Bloodwise
www.bloodwise.org.uk

Beating Bowel Cancer
www.beatingbowelcancer.org

Bowel Cancer UK
www.bowelcanceruk.org.uk

The Brain Tumour Charity
www.thebraintumourcharity.org

Breast Cancer Care
www.breastcancercare.org.uk

Breast Cancer Now
www.breastcancernow.org

CoppaFeel!
www.coppafeel.org

The Eve Appeal
www.eveappeal.org.uk

Jo's Cervical Cancer Trust
www.jostrust.org.uk

Movember Foundation
www.uk.movember.com

Prostate Cancer UK
www.prostatecanceruk.org

Children and Young Adults

Clic Sargent
www.clicsargent.org.uk

Shine Cancer Support
www.shinecancersupport.org

Teenage Cancer Trust
www.teenagecancertrust.org

Trekstock
www.trekstock.com

Clinical Trials

www.cancerresearchuk.org/about-cancer/find-a-clinical-trial

Support and Health

About Herbs (run by Sloan Kettering)
www.aboutherbs.com

British Acupuncture Council
www.acupuncture.org.uk

British Nutrition Foundation
www.nutrition.org.uk

Girl vs Cancer
www.girlvscancer.co.uk

Give blood
www.blood.co.uk

Look Good Feel Better
www.lookgoodfeelbetter.co.uk

Mind
www.mind.org.uk

Race for Life
www.raceforlife.cancerresearch.uk.org

Online and Apps

@Bowelbabe
www.instagram.com/bowelbabe
www.facebook.com/bowelbabe
www.twitter.com/bowelbabe

#fuckyoucancer

NHS Couch to 5km App
www.nhs.co.uk/live-well/exercise/get-running-with-couch-
to-5km

Things Cancer Made Me Say
www.thesun.co.uk/topic/things-cancer-made-me-say

You, Me and the Big C – Podcast
www.bbc.co.uk/youmebigc

Bloggers in the Club!

Alice May Purkiss
www.alicemaypurkiss.co.uk

Almost Amazing Grace
www.almostamazinggrace.co.uk

Beneath the Weather
www.beneaththeweather.com

Better Fools
www.betterfools.com

Big C Little Me
www.bigclittleme.co.uk

Bonnie H Fox
www.twitter.com/bonniehfox

Brenda Won't Back Down
www.brendawontbackdown.com

Cancer with a Smile
www.cancerwithasmile.com

Hiking Boots and Killer Heels
www.hikingbootsandkillerheels.wordpress.com

How to Glitter a Turd
www.howtoglitteraturd.com

Lucy's Melanoma Adventure
www.Lucysmelanomaadventure.wordpress.com

Me and My Four
www.meandmyfour.com

Melanoma Jo
www.melanomajo.com

Acknowledgements

I find it incredible that out of the whole book, I have procrastinated longest over writing my thankyous! I didn't want to cock it up, offend anyone or basically forget (due to chemo brain!) any of the amazing people who have gone above and beyond to help me. I find that each time I try to write this, I end up bawling my eyes out like a big pussy, reaching for the wine and then passing out saying 'another day!' One shot, Deborah, one shot at thanking those you love – and knowing me I'll end up giving the most thanks to Winston my dog (who is bloody awesome to say the least) for being literally always at my side. But here goes...

Shit – I just mentioned the dog first! But Sebastien, my darling husband, I do love you more. Thank you for being my rock, for holding me – and everything around me – together when it's falling down. Thank you for being there at 3am when I'm crying and for holding my hand, or not holding my hand if I'm in shut down mode and grumpy! Thank you for taking everything I throw at you and coming back with unconditional love. Thank you for always supporting and guiding me in whatever wild adventure I wake up and decide to pursue. It breaks my heart that I most likely won't be able to see our kids grow old. But, whilst I may never come to terms with that idea, knowing they have you as a father will make the whole thing just a little easier. Please care for our babies and know how much I love you and am proud of you – always.

Thank you to the incredible medical team who keep me alive so I'm able to spend one more day enjoying life. To Professor David Cunningham and the team at the Royal Marsden. Thank you for your relentless drive that not only keeps me ticking, but ensures that I and many others will benefit from the latest research in cancer prevention and cure. I'm blown away by your passion in working to get the best outcomes for every person and for your relentless patience with my million and one questions and weekly moments of panic attacks / freak outs / throwing toys out of the pram. The day I found out I had stage 4 bowel cancer, you called me to say that 'whilst it was a shock' you guaranteed to do whatever was humanly possible to keep me alive, kitchen sink and all. It was the best bloody thing anyone could have said to me in the darkest moment of my life. I have utter faith that you and the team will do your best and I'm hoping that your work and some good luck will enable us to kick this can far along the road!

Writing a book published by Penguin was a pipe dream that I thought could only happen to other people. Thank you to Sam Jackson for plucking me out of obscurity, for giving me a shot at proving we could do something new in the market and for having my back even when I missed every single deadline going, to the point that I considered using 'the dog ate it' as an excuse! Thank you Penguin Random House for taking me under your wing – it's a total privilege to be an author with you. As a child your books lined my bookshelves and I'd fall asleep always wondering what it would feel like to write a book with you. Now I know that it feels incredible and it's something of which I'm so proud.

Thank you to Adelaide Leeder for bringing the writing to life through your incredible illustrations. I could not have wished for a better match and I'm so happy I found you.

To my incredible friends from all walks of life, who have laughed with me, cried with me, got drunk with me, come to chemo with me, sent death jokes to me, fed me, sorted my kids out for me and generally acted as incredible rocks for me and my family, thank you for allowing us to focus on one thing – living! Thank you for bringing light and laughter into a place where at times it is dark. And thank you for lifting us up, wiping our tears and arming us with wine, good food, incredible love and friendship and amazing memories.

To Deborah Alsina and the amazing team at Bowel Cancer UK, thank you for all you do to raise awareness that you are never too young to have bowel cancer. And yes – one day we will stop it. Thank you for the support you have shown to me and the entire network of patients and families who value the work you do every day very much.

To David Mellville, my bowel surgeon – I could not have asked for a kinder medical expert to get me through the initial shock. Thank you for knowing that when I said I needed mashed potato and red wine, I really did need it!

Thank you so much to Steph Douglas, Emma Campbell, Brenda Trenowden, Rhiannon Bradley, Stacey Heale, Athena Lamnisos and Audrey Allan for sharing your stories for the book with such honesty. Thank you for all you do in continuing to raise awareness so that others know they are not alone.

Justine Paine – you have made me realise the power of writing. Thank you for each and every note you wrote to me since my diagnosis. Your act of kindness touched me and lifted me more than you will ever imagine.

To the Fuck Cancer Club (FCC) girls and my online Instagram family. Thank you for the love, support and for totally getting what I feel like. I know you have my back and together we've got this shit!

To my 'You, Me and the Big C' podcast family at BBC Radio 5 Live – Rachael Bland, Lauren Mahon, Mike 'the bear' Holt and Al Entwistle – thank you. You have provided hope, friendship and an incredible bond that only hours on trains, in studios and talking honestly about poo emoji costumes at funerals could do!

To Keith Poole and Lizzie Parry, my *Sun* online crew, thank you for always having my back, for guiding and supporting me and for giving me the best home to talk about shit! I'm so proud to be a '*Sun girl*'. Thankfully for our readers I kept my tits under wraps!

To my mum and dad. I'm gutted you have to watch me go through this but thank you for the unconditional love and relentless support you give to Sebastien, me and the kids. If I die, I know the kids prefer you anyway! Sarah and Ben, I would still pick you as brother and sister even if I had a choice. Thank you for everything, but one bit of advice bro: remember dad is bald. Genetics. That's all I'm saying!

Hugo and Eloise, you are my world. You are my everything and I love you beyond comprehension. Know that whatever happens I'm with you, I'm at your side and I believe you can do anything you want to do. I'm so proud of you and all I ask for you in life is to make the most of every single day. To love hard, take risks, find something you are passionate about, do it well and have no regrets. I don't. How can I when I have you in my life.

Love Deborah X

Index